NATURAL
FLEXIBILITY

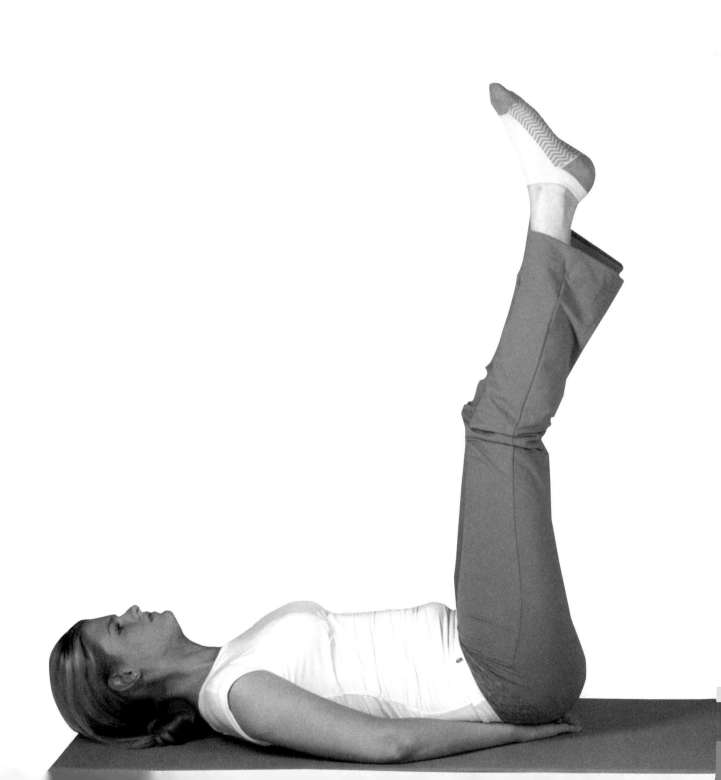

NATURAL FLEXIBILITY

The New Risk-Free
Alternative to Stretching

By CHARLES KENNY, MD

PHOTOGRAPHS *by* AYDIN ARJOMAND

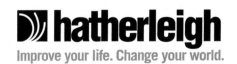

Improve your life. Change your world.

))) hatherleigh

5–22 46th Avenue, Suite 200
Long Island City, NY 11101
www.hatherleighpress.com

Hatherleigh Press is committed to preserving and protecting the natural resources of the Earth. Environmentally responsible and sustainable practices are embraced within the company's mission statement.

Hatherleigh Press is a member of the Publishers Earth Alliance, committed to preserving and protecting the natural resources of the planet while developing a sustainable business model for the book publishing industry.

PEA Member   Recycled Content   Earth-Friendly Printing

Earth-Friendly Printing: The interior of this book was printed with soy ink.

Recycled Content: This book is printed on 17% recycled paper, made up of 7% Pre and 10% Post Consumer Waste.

Library of Congress Cataloging-in-Publication Data
Kenny, Charles, M.D.
Natural flexibility : the complete guide to resistance stretching for golf, tennis, running, sports and fitness / Charles Kenny.
p. cm.
ISBN 978–1–57826–284–7 (pbk. : alk. paper)   1. Physical education and training.
2. Stretching exercises.   I. Title.
GV711.5.K46 2008
613.7'182—dc22
2008037043

All Hatherleigh Press titles are available for bulk purchase, special promotions, and premiums. For more information, please contact the manager of our Special Sales Department at 1-800-367-2550

Interior design by Maria Mendez
Cover design by Howard Grossman, 12E DESIGN
Neuwirth & Associates, Inc.

To Jeremy, Sam, and of course,
Barbara, and to my Mom.

ACKNOWLEDGEMENTS

A BOOK SUCH as *Natural Flexibility* makes its way into reality through the efforts of many people. An author can only claim a portion of the responsibility. Still, there are those whose contributions along the way have been so crucial that the book would not exist without them. One person in particular, my wife, Barbara, is undeniably such a contributor. This book was born and first showed signs of life through her labor. She has nurtured and protected it every step of the way. Thank you, Barbara. My two sons, Sam and Jeremy, kept me going with encouragement and their constantly good spirits, helping equally on both sides of the camera and computer. Special thanks go from me to Diane and Peter for recognizing the potential of "Don't Stretch" and giving it a leg up early on.

I am also grateful to many medical and exercise professionals, as well as athletes and dancers, who remain nameless here, who coached me as I struggled to untie the knot of confusion that binds stretching to the world of sport, dance, and exercise.

Sandy McNay, Leigh-Ellen Figueroa, and Barbara deserve recognition for the photographic and photogenic support they bring to the book.

Of course, the Hatherleigh team, especially June and Anna, drew back the final curtain as *Natural Flexibility* stepped forward from the imaginary to the real. In particular, I know that Andrew pulled the right rabbit out of the hat.

Charles Kenny, M.D.
September 2008

Contents

MY GOAL IS to teach a new flexibility for dedicated athletes and dancers, for their trainers and coaches, and for anyone who strives to improve fitness and performance.

Natural flexibility is not really new, because the human body already achieves a certain amount of flexibility instinctively through techniques like the ones you will find in this book. But this natural flexibility is new to the world of exercise, sport, and dance because it has been confused with stretching.

At first glance, the exercises that improve natural flexibility even look like stretching, but the body is doing something completely different. The dedicated athlete and dancer will soon realize that this new flexibility is much better. Why? Because this natural flexibility truly improves performance. This natural flexibility really prevents injuries. It relieves soreness and tightness when soreness and tightness are not serious, and when it doesn't, *Natural Flexibility* will tell you what to do next. Additionally, natural flexibility is the natural way to wake up. A few minutes at the beginning of each day revitalizes your body and mind and helps prevent common low back and neck pain.

The foundation of *Natural Flexibility* is progressive sequential isometric exercise, or *PSI* (pronounced "sigh"). PSI is based on your body's natural isometric muscular contractions. You use these contractions all day long, and especially at the ultimate limits of your range of motion during athletics and dance. The end of a pitcher's windup and the backswing of a golfer's drive or a tennis serve are common examples of the body's instinctive use of isometric exercise.

Your body also uses isometric exercises to wake you up. Common English usage calls this spontaneous isometric exercise "stretching," but your body is asking you to do something much different from what they tell you to do in stretching books. Check this for yourself. When you wake and "stretch," does your body "relax with the stretch" or tighten your muscles? *Natural Flexibility* will turn your thinking all around. I will show you how to take almost any relaxed stretch and convert it into an Ultimate *PSI*. Ultimate *PSI* develops natural flexibility for peak performance at the extreme limit of range of motion, just where you used to stretch.

Coaches and teachers responsible for the instruction and safety of others should take the time to become familiar with *PSI*. *PSI* is founded on the most up-to-date principles of injury prevention and performance enhancement. And *PSI* is easy to do, without any special equipment, anywhere stretching used to be done. *PSI* can be used to evaluate soreness and pain in the athlete and dancer and help answer the recurring questions "How bad is the injury?" and "How much can the athlete safely do?" In addition, with *Natural Flexibility* test results in hand, it will be easy for coaches to identify muscle overuse patterns and pinpoint underlying flaws in the athlete's technique. Certified athletic trainers and physical therapists will find *PSI* invaluable to formulate treatment plans and assist in functional evaluations to determine the rate of progression of exercise during rehabilitation. As scientific evidence accumulates that stretching has doubtful benefits and may be harmful, trainers and coaches frequently find themselves at a loss for what to recommend to dedicated athletes to improve flexibility and warm up. With *Natural Flexibility*, it is easy to maximize dynamic flexibility and avoid the risks and performance impairments of stretching.

Yes, I am telling you not to stretch. Throw out your stretching books. For natural flexibility, you need *Natural Flexibility*.

CHARLES KENNY, M.D.
Fellow, American Academy of Orthopaedic Surgeons
Fellow, American College of Sports Medicine

THE
SCIENCE OF
NATURAL
FLEXIBILITY

Chapter 1

The Fundamentals of Flexibility

ATHLETES AND DANCERS realize that flexibility is the foundation of fitness, performance, and injury prevention, but just what is flexibility? Is all flexibility the same? What is the best kind of flexibility for you? In spite of the crucial importance of flexibility to exercise and well-being, the answers to these questions are commonly buried under myths, misunderstandings and false assumptions. This chapter will teach you the truth about flexibility.

WHAT IS FLEXIBILITY?

Almost everyone agrees that flexibility is an indicator of fitness. But when we use the word "flexibility," are we all thinking of the same thing? The American College of Sports Medicine's 2006 *Guidelines for Exercise Testing and Prescription* says, "Flexibility is the ability to move a joint through its complete range of motion." The President's Council on Physical Fitness and Sports cites Holt's definition of flexibility: "the intrinsic property of body tissues, which determines the range of motion achievable without injury at a joint or group of joints." Most of you would agree that one of these definitions is something like what you have in mind when you think of flexibility.

When you read scientific papers about flexibility, the titles, abstracts, and often the main bodies of the papers use the unqualified word "flexibility." This conjures up the above concepts and inferred associations with ease of motion, fitness, and injury prevention. Nevertheless, the kind of flexibility studied outside the laboratory is *almost never* the flexibility just defined. Rather, "flexibility" as typically evaluated by scientific clinical studies is a limited kind of flexibility called *static flexibility*. Static flexibility is defined by the subject's ability to tolerate a passive stretch; that is, a measured stretch, while the subject relaxes the muscles being stretched. Unlike the President's Council's definition, the definition of static flexibility does not specifically include injury avoidance. Strictly speaking, it has nothing to do with the ability of a joint to move, either. Static flexibility reflects only the limit of passive motion. Static flexibility demands, for its proper assessment, that the muscle undergoing evaluation relaxes completely.

This relaxed kind of flexibility, the kind measured by and created by stretching, has absolutely no place in the dynamic world of sport and fitness. Stretching advocates have been selling stretching to athletes and dancers on the false pretense that relaxed muscles are the best and only alternative to tight muscles. This is absolutely untrue. During physical exercise, your muscles are activated and controlled by your brain and your spinal nerves through messages carried to and from your muscles, tendons, and joints. These muscles are not relaxed. Yet every athlete and dancer already knows that these warmed-up, activated muscles do not feel tight. These activated muscles are your best alternative to tight muscles. Activated muscles *feel relaxed*, but they are not. They set the stage for peak performance, decreased risk of injury, and maximum flexibility. We will take a closer look at a new definition for flexibility, one based on activated instead of relaxed muscles, in chapter 2. Then, we will look at specific exercises designed to activate your muscles and joints.

FLEXIBILITY AND FITNESS

Intuitively, your concept of flexibility as an important component of fitness automatically leads you to suspect that more flexibility is better than less. But, if you are going to judge the value of your flexibility by how much you can stretch your relaxed muscles, you are in for some surprises. Did you know that after reviewing 361 scientific articles, the United States Center for Disease Control found no basis for the claim that stretching decreases risk of injury? Coaches and trainers frequently encourage stretching to increase flexibility because decreased static flexibility has been related to increased injuries in athletes and military personnel. But decreased flexibility due to muscular tightness is a normal protective response, so cause and effect in such cases are easy to confuse. The assumption is usually made that decreased flexibility caused the injuries, but actually, undiagnosed conditions may have been present that not only caused decreased flexibility, but also predisposed to injury. Assumptions about flexibility are commonly made about performance and fitness as well. But just because decreased flexibility has been correlated to some physical quality does not mean that decreased flexibility is the cause, or that stretching will turn things around. To see this clearly, consider this: It is known that men are less flexible than women. It would be ridiculous to conclude that decreased flexibility causes you to be male, or that stretching to increase your flexibility will make you female.

Doesn't this raise serious questions about the reliability of the static flexibility as a fitness concept?

THE ORIGINS OF DOUBT

In medical school, I learned that stretching was essential to prevent injuries. But, one afternoon in Baltimore in 1978, while I was assisting the team physician for the Orioles during my training in orthopaedic surgery, a player came limping into the clinic unable to put any weight on his leg. The trainer helped him onto the exam table as the player told us how he had been hurt: he hit a line drive by third base, started for first, felt a shot in his leg, and fell to the ground. Once he was in position on the exam table, I could see that his leg was grossly swollen and discolored. He could not exert any downward pressure with his foot, and I could feel a big indentation where his Achilles tendon was supposed to be. He had ruptured the tendon. He turned to the trainer and asked, "Hey, I think I hurt my leg *while I was stretching*—is that possible?"

A few years later, when I was on call for dance injuries at Jacob's Pillow in the Berkshires in western Massachusetts, I was asked to see a dancer who was hurt and had to go on that evening. He gave me this account of the injury: He had been stretching as usual when he felt a burning pain high in his upper thigh, in the back near his buttock. The pain grew worse as he continued, even though he was "being extra careful." He stopped stretching, got up, and tried what he thought was a very simple jump. He felt the burning area rip apart. He could not bear any weight on the leg after that. On examination, I found a big hole high in the back of his thigh under his buttock where his hamstring tendon was supposed to attach to the pelvic ischial bone (the bone you sit on). The tendon had totally pulled off from the bone.

Through the years, many of my patients have insisted that they were injured during their regular stretching routine or shortly thereafter. They had followed the rules: they stretched "correctly," slowly, carefully, not too fast. Still, they got hurt. It became clear to me that stretching was not as safe or effective as it was supposed to be. At the same time, I suspected that hamstring stretching was not helping the increasing number of severe knee ligament injuries in already-flexible female soccer and basketball players. Nevertheless, many of these injured athletes and dancers went back to stretching because they had no other warm-up or flexibility routine to follow.

FLEXIBILITY WITHOUT STRETCHING

Natural Flexibility will introduce you to *PSI*, which includes much better exercises than stretching and makes you feel good without the risk. My method will give you:

- Exercises to warm up for any sport or fitness activity
- Exercises to increase flexibility, strength, balance, and fitness and to decrease injuries
- Ultimate *PSI* to maximize dynamic flexibility for specific sports and dance, and a way to turn almost any relaxed stretch into Ultimate *PSI*
- Exercises to wake up in the morning
- Exercises for when you're sore, that tell you what is wrong, why it's happening, what you can and can't do with it, and what to do about it. Once you learn to use it, you can take your *Natural Flexibility* test results to your coach, pro, trainer, or therapist to help them pinpoint what you need.
- Exercises specific to alleviating and preventing neck and back pain, the most common types of pain associated with regular physical activity

The wake-up exercises will give you a new energy and refreshed posture all day long. The warm ups will prepare you for sports and fitness training, as well as test all the sore spots. I have selected exercises to work every major muscle group and joint in your body without wasting your time with duplication. After having spent over 30 years repairing and rehabilitating damaged and broken bodies, I am pleased to recommend *PSI*, based on natural, instinctive exercises, specifically designed to replace harmful stretches that often lead to soreness or injury. *PSI* not only comes through where stretching fails, *PSI* helps figure out what your body is telling you when you have pain and what to do about it. Ultimate *PSI* is for the millions of earnest athletes and dancers who innocently subject themselves to risks every time they stretch to improve their flexibility.

MUSCLE HARMONY

Simply put, muscles are your body's tools of self-expression. Within your body, thousands of muscle fibers await your command. A series of reflexes and a complex network of nerve connections tweak and adjust how each muscle fiber contracts, so the muscle can do exactly what you ordered in a harmonious, coordinated way. Your muscle fibers will try to do anything you ask.

In fact, it is so easy to command your faithful muscles that you often make them do things they should not really do.

We'll talk more about that later. But for now, let's look closer at the relationship between your muscles and flexibility.

DYNAMIC FLEXIBILITY AND MUSCLE BALANCE

Muscles work in teams, like horses pulling a stage coach, to create something called *dynamic flexibility*. The main muscles that pull like horses, are called the *agonists*. You move your body with your agonist muscles. More importantly, you slow down, steer, and control the specific nuances of your body's movement with your *antagonist* muscles, the same way a stage coach rider pulls back on the reins to slow, turn, or stop the team of horses.

Let's look at an example. When you swing a golf club, it is the *agonist* muscles in your shoulder that move your arm so you can force the club forward to hit the ball. During the follow-through, it is the *antagonist* muscles that slow your arm down.

Note that the follow-through is critical: you need to give the antagonist muscles time to slow down smoothly and bring the action to a halt so the supporting tissues in the shoulder joint and arm are not damaged. Otherwise, you will incur injury.

If you perform the motion in reverse, such as during a backswing motion, the muscles switch roles: the antagonists become the agonists and *vice versa*.

TIGHTNESS AND SORENESS

How do injuries happen? Well, we have a tendency to make our muscles do things they really shouldn't do. For example, you command your muscles to help you to sit in awkward positions for hours at a time. You make them swing a golf club even when they are exhausted. You ask them to sprint for first base when you haven't warmed up. You force them to swing a tennis racquet improperly as you practice your serve with bad technique.

What is the result? Often, these abused muscles become *tight* and *sore*.

Muscle *tightness* and *soreness* are signs of overused and improperly used muscles—the result of a malfunction in the way the nerves control the muscles, leading to loss of muscle harmony. Some muscle fibers become tighter than others. In short, the uncomfortable feelings of tightness and soreness are signs that your muscles are not working together in the way they should.

This discomfort is also a two-part warning. Not only is your body telling you that you did something wrong, it is also warning that if continue the same pattern, or try something harder, things could get worse.

The antagonist muscles are frequently injured or overpowered because not only is the job they do more difficult, but these muscles are often ignored in warm up and strengthening routines. If your antagonist muscles are weak, or if damage is occurring because they cannot control an action, your body will make these antagonist muscles tight to protect you.

What *Not* to Do

Of course, you already know what the stretching gurus would tell you to do for tight antagonist muscles: Stretch the tight muscles! But this is a short-sighted approach and yet another example of why stretching, as commonly defined, does you more harm than good.

After you stretch, you will surely notice that your muscles feel less tight. For one thing, stretching increases static flexibility (we'll look closer at how in chapter 2). But this will only last for a few minutes. And, because stretching also has deactivated the tight muscles, your newly relaxed muscles won't be in control the way they should be, and you have actually made your situation worse. That is, if you were to go ahead and use your body as though everything were okay, you would have decreased control because of stretching. On top of that, whatever problem was originally making the antagonists muscles tight would now get worse.

You have to stop this pattern. Because your body learns to do everything you practice, in exactly the position you practiced it, every time you stretch as part of your training, you are training your muscles to relax and do nothing in positions where you need them most.

ISOMETRICS—A CINDERELLA STORY

The goals of stretching and increased flexibility can be achieved almost entirely with isometrics. However, scientific studies of these two "step-sisters" usually do not acknowledge this fact. For starters, *isometric exercise increases static flexibility just as much as stretching*. Isometric exercise not only activates muscles, it teaches them to activate more quickly and powerfully. Indeed, over time, isometric exercise increases strength much more effectively than stretching, *plus* the degree of difficulty and length of time spent on isometric exercise can be adjusted according to desired goals. Also, isometrics have been found to function as a satisfactory warm up in reducing injuries. Isometrics have other benefits. They make you feel good. They relieve pain and stiffness. They help adjust blood flow in preparation for getting out of bed. This is particularly valuable for patients who have been bedridden after surgery or injuries. Isometrics have even been shown to lower blood pressure in people with hypertension, and some studies suggest they can decrease the desire to smoke cigarettes.

Isometrics are natural exercises. That is, your body naturally engages in isometric exercises all day long. When you reach for a glass of water, your body uses an isometric contraction to hold the glass. When you stand still, your body uses isometric contractions to hold your head and body in one place. When you yawn and "stretch," your body uses isometric contractions—not the relaxed stretches you learn about in stretching manuals! When you jump, or throw a ball, or at the endpoint of your stride as you sprint, your body uses isometric contractions at the places in the range of motion where the movement changes direction.

With isometrics, you also avoid many of the pitfalls of relaxed, static stretching. That is, unlike relaxed stretching, isometric exercises do not repress muscular activity or create conflicting learning patterns for muscles near the extremes of joint motion. And isometrics, unlike relaxed stretching, do not require an extreme of range of motion to increase flexibility.

Why Isometrics are Confused with Stretching

During an isometric contraction, muscle length does not change and the joint does not move. For this reason, isometrics are often confused with relaxed stretching; that is, because they look alike.

Unfortunately, this confusion often creeps into supposedly scientific studies that group relaxed stretching and isometrics together, and so whatever benefits are discovered are claimed to be a sole result of "stretching." This is extremely misleading and serves to reinforce erroneous conclusions and recommendations, because coaches and trainers are led to believe that benefits are due entirely to the relaxed stretching recommended in stretching books.

It is likewise common for advocates of stretching to point to the spontaneous "stretching" of a cat to emphasize the (supposedly) natural aspects of relaxed stretching. In reality, a cat is performing an isometric exercise because muscular activity, without joint motion, is clearly visible during the action. Next time you feel the urge to yawn and "stretch," prove this for yourself. Instead of going with your natural instinct to tighten all your muscles, "relax with the stretch" as the stretching-book gurus tell you to do. You will see how unfulfilling and unnatural a relaxed stretch really is. The whole purpose of the natural isometric exercise that we commonly call a "stretch" is to tighten muscles during the action, not to relax them as in an artificially contrived, static stretch. If we really wanted to "relax" when we stretched, we would stretch to help us fall asleep, not to help us wake up!

The tendency for common English usage to call a natural isometric exercise a "stretch" should not be a reason to mislead dedicated athletes and dancers into performing the worthless and potentially harmful relaxed-stretch exercises commonly found in stretching manuals.

Chapter 2

A Breakthrough *to* Natural Flexibility

BY NOW YOU'VE surely gotten the idea that natural flexibility is the kind of flexibility you want: Flexibility you can count on to improve performance . . . flexibility that will prevent injury . . . flexibility that makes you feel *great*. Natural flexibility is also easily implemented into your exercise, sport, or dance routines and can provide a guide to what you can safely do when you take your workout to the next level. Natural flexibility is surprisingly easy to obtain. In fact, your body already has it. This chapter will teach you how to maximize your own natural flexibility.

A NEW FLEXIBILITY

We have already learned that flexibility is generally defined as "the ability of a joint to move through a full range of motion." We have also learned why this definition is in fact very limited, and is often used to justify worthless—and often harmful—stretching techniques that are based on the false assumption that "more relaxed flexibility equals better flexibility." Even worse, we have seen how it is common to access flexibility by stretching, and we have learned how traditional stretching, because it often does in fact help individuals to increase static flexibility, is misleading and can lead to a self-perpetuating loop of misunderstanding. Stretching gurus would have you believe that *how flexible you are* is determined by *how far you can stretch your relaxed body*. This overly simple mechanical assessment fails to consider the *dynamic* aspects of performance and injury prevention.

I define flexibility as *the ability of a properly prepared joint or series of joints to move or be moved with control and safety through a range of motion appropriate for the optimal performance of an activity to be undertaken.*

Put more simply, your flexibility should be measured against *what you intend to do, after you warm up.*

Flexibility should not be determined by how much you can move flaccid, numb muscles while you "relax" during a stretch. Flexibility should depend on your activated nervous system as much as your warmed-up, well-trained body. Flexibility gives you the power to train for performance and agility. Whether you are aware of it or not, you are reflexively, instantaneously modifying your flexibility during your sport or dance by adjusting how tightly your muscles will contract while you perform. This fast-paced gear shifting relies on strength, control, and training. This is *dynamic flexibility*, the kind of flexibility you really want. Forget about the relaxed, "falling-asleep" flexibility of stretching!

ISOMETRIC EXERCISE: ADVANTAGES OVER STRETCHING

While isometric exercise looks a lot like stretching, the effects of isometric exercise are totally different from the effects of stretching. Stretching advocates take advantage of the superficial similarities of isometric exercise and stretching, making stretching seem better to the world of sport and dance than it actually is. Because you have probably been exposed to that (misguided) "school" of stretching in your own life already, it is important to take a look at what really happens when you follow the typical stretching manual's instructions to stretch, in comparison to what happens during isometric exercises.

Viscoelasticity

When you stretch a rubber band, it lengthens in proportion to how much force you apply. This is because the rubber band is an elastic material. Living tissues are not this simple.

Living tissues, such as muscles, tendons, and joints, are viscoelastic. That is, when you stretch a muscle, it becomes more flexible, because the stretching squeezes water out of the muscle, tendon, and joint, causing long molecules to slide past one another and change shape, which ultimately lengthens the muscle. This process takes a few minutes to occur, but once it happens, the muscle and tendon are more flexible.

Surprisingly, this effect usually only lasts a few minutes, depending on how much time you took to stretch, because the tissues quickly reabsorb the water, and the molecules automatically return to their original shapes. Among other things, this means that you must remain active to preserve the viscoelasticity effects of stretching. Furthermore, stretching is customarily performed with the joint in only one, extreme position, so stretching does not increase flexibility in other places in the joint's range of motion. This is because when you stretch and pressure is applied to a joint while it is in a fixed position, fluid is squeezed from the contact areas only on the opposing joint surfaces and only from the ligaments and other supporting structures that come under stress during the stretch. Since fluid is not being squeezed from areas of the joint surface that are not in contact during the stretch, nor is fluid being squeezed from the supporting structures, these areas are not addressed. In short, the ligaments and capsule that stabilize your joint through its entire range of motion, as well as the majority of joint surface itself that you rely on for smooth movement, are all completely ignored by stretching. What kind of warm up is that?

Isometric exercises increase viscoelasticity in the same ways as stretching, but because isometrics can be applied at different places in the joint's range of motion, they are a much more logical approach to joint preparation for sport or exercise.

Muscle Relaxation

We've seen how viscoelasticity is influenced by stretching. The other main and much misunderstood effect of stretching on the body is muscle relaxation.

To effectively partake in a traditional stretch, the subject must willfully inhibit any contraction of the stretched muscle. That is why, in stretching manuals, the authors will always tell you to "relax with the stretch." However, this is potentially dangerous and counterproductive. Why? Because regular relaxed stretching teaches muscles to relax at the *endpoints* in the range of motion—right when muscle activation is most critical!

Endpoints of range of motion are places where joints, muscles and tendons are most vulnerable because rapid decelerations and accelerations occur as the direction of motion changes.

At these extreme lengths, muscle strength is diminished and leverage can magnify unexpected or excessive forces. Activities such as golf, tennis, running, baseball, and dance regularly and repeatedly put the joints in these extreme positions. In order to avoid injury and maximize performance, the body relies on precise muscular control of the motion.

Flexibility training that employs regularly repeated stretching exercises over many weeks—like any other training technique—will program motor memory. This motor memory is specific to the place in the arc of motion at which the training occurs. That is, the way muscles are used during a stretch will tend to repeat itself later, in the middle of a series of movements. If muscles are taught to relax during a stretch at critical endpoints of range of motion, that same pattern of relaxation will resurface during an exercise or a routine when the critical endpoint is reached. In other words, when definitive muscle contraction and control are most needed, the negative training experience of stretching discourages your muscles from engaging properly! Stretching routines repeatedly conflict with other training techniques because stretching practice trains muscles to relax.

Isometric exercise has exactly the opposite effect of stretching on muscle activation. That is why, at the endpoints of range of motion, where motion changes direction, your body already uses isometric muscular contractions naturally to control the storage and retrieval of muscle and tendon energy. This energy storage and retrieval is essential for peak performance and only happens with well-controlled muscle activation. For instance, at the endpoint of a backswing, windup, or follow-through, or the low point in a gymnastic or ballet split, your body naturally uses isometric muscular contractions. Your muscles do *not* "relax," as is recommended by many stretching gurus, at the endpoint of a sport or dance movement. In fact, if these maneuvers were repeatedly attempted with relaxed muscles, not only would power and control suffer, but serious injuries would also occur.

Another thing to keep in mind is, when a muscle is relaxed, it only absorbs about half as much energy before tearing as it would while it was contracting. So, from an injury prevention standpoint, at the vulnerable extreme of length, it is much better to train a muscle to contract with an isometric exercise, than to relax with a static stretch.

ISOMETRICS IN ACTION

Amazingly, isometric exercise makes you stronger almost immediately. This miraculous effect is the result of immediate improvement in the way your nerves control your muscles. Isometric contractions increase the speed and efficiency by which your nerves activate your muscles.

Isometric exercise also increases your flexibility immediately, to the same degree that stretching does—but does not come at the cost of flabby, limp muscles, as with stretching. Instead, isometric exercise gives you flexibility with improved strength and dynamic control. This is why cats don't stretch when they wake up; they do isometrics. (Sorry, gurus.)

Proprioceptive neuromuscular facilitation (PNF) stretching combines a relaxed static stretch with isometric exercise. PNF stretching is of special interest to exercise professionals because it lessens the drawbacks of static stretching while it enhances the flexibility effects. The more isometrics used, the greater the PNF-stretching flexibility effect. *The underappreciated aspect of PNF stretching is the isometric component.* Indeed, the benefits of the isometric exercise component of PNF stretching more than make up for the negative effects of static-stretch training. (Those of you who know only a little about PNF stretching should be especially careful not to confuse it with Ultimate *PSI.*)

EARN YOUR FLEXIBILITY WITH *PSI*

PSI, progressive sequential isometric exercise (pronounced "sigh") turns on, tests, and maintains your body.

How does *PSI* promote a much more dynamic flexibility than stretching? *PSI* prepares and activates the spine, arms, and legs, but it is not just restricted to the muscles. *PSI* also prepares and activates the joints, ligaments, tendons, blood vessels, and nervous system—all at the same time. It is important to note that, although *PSI* can look like stretching if the joint is near an extreme range of motion, the effects of these isometric exercises differ greatly from those of stretching.

PSI is isometric exercise repeated with increasing amounts of effort at one place in the range of motion. Next, the same exercises are repeated at new places within the normal joint range of motion, in increased degrees of joint flexion and extension, to increase strength and flexibility. You can do an isometric exercise in any position you want, but you should start in an easy position to warm up. Unless it is preceded by a proper warm up, *any* exercise done in an extreme position puts the body in jeopardy. You will soon see how *PSI* is the natural and logical way to warm up.

PSI further increases flexibility by working each joint from different angles, starting in the mid-range of motion and working toward the extremes, so the ligaments, cartilage, and other joint structures become as flexible as possible without risk or discomfort.

The progressive nature of *PSI* ensures that effort is in proportion to flexibility. In other words, with *PSI*, you start very easy and only do more if you are able. At the lowest levels of effort, gentle *PSI* is the best warm-up for sore or injured muscles and joints. At the same time that you increase your flexibility, *PSI* helps you to figure out if you are really ready to tackle a vigorous activity. *PSI* also helps you to determine how vigorous you can be without getting hurt. *PSI* increases flexibility, strength, and control immediately and also over time. First, improved blood flow and faster muscle activation bring about an immediate increase in flexibility and strength. As weeks pass, training effects lead to gains in structural strength and neuromuscular control. You will have earned your flexibility with *PSI*.

Ultimate *PSI*

Ultimate *PSI*, like *PSI*, is meant to increase flexibility benefits without the risks of stretching, but Ultimate *PSI* is done at the maximum flexibility position.

The limit of a joint's range of motion is the place where action reverses and energy is transferred; in other words, it refers to the furthest limit your body wants to go. The windup of a pitch, the backswing of a forehand, the follow-through of a golf swing, and the countermovement dip in preparation for a jump all have one thing in common: the storage and retrieval of energy. Momentum of motion is stored as potential energy in the tendons and ligaments and released back as momentum once again to combine with the energy of contraction of the muscles. Normally, this energy transfer relies on precisely controlled natural isometric muscle contractions to maximize power and decrease harmful stresses. Stretching trains muscles to give up at this most crucial place in the action.

Ultimate *PSI* uses natural isometric muscle contractions, exactly the kind your body uses at the ultimate reach in the windup of a pitch or the bottom of the dip just before you leap in the air. Ultimate *PSI* achieves the same viscoelastic flexibility increases as stretching, but the dynamic natural flexibility training effects of Ultimate *PSI* far outclass those of stretching.

Let's look more closely at a common stretch for the left shoulder and arm (on the left) and compare it with an Ultimate *PSI*.

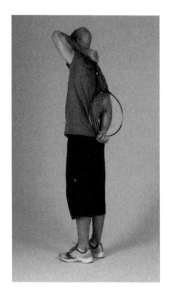
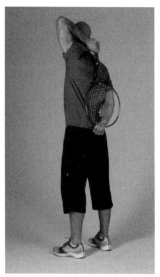

Hmmm. They look the same. We have to do better than that.

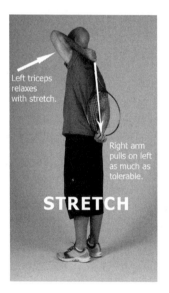
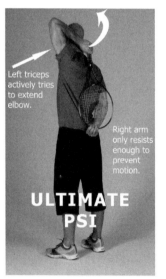

Left triceps relaxes with stretch.

Right arm pulls on left as much as tolerable.

STRETCH

Left triceps actively tries to extend elbow.

Right arm only resists enough to prevent motion.

ULTIMATE PSI

Let's look at the differences between the stretch and Ultimate *PSI* for the left arm and left shoulder.

1. In the stretch, all the muscles in the left shoulder and arm are relaxed.
   In Ultimate *PSI*, all the muscles of the left shoulder are contracting.
2. In the stretch, the left arm is doing nothing.
   In Ultimate *PSI*, the left arm is trying to pull the right hand up.

3. In the stretch, the right arm is trying to pull the left hand down.

In Ultimate *PSI*, the right hand is resisting just enough to prevent any movement from occurring.

Any stretch can be turned into an Ultimate *PSI* if you resist the stretch so no movement occurs.

TRUST YOUR BODY

If your hamstrings are tight, what is your body trying to tell you? Although stretching dogma leads us to believe that tight muscles can simply be corrected by stretching, muscle tightness actually means something—your body is trying to communicate with you. In many instances, your body is telling you that you simply need to warm up before you can expect to achieve the motion you want. Or perhaps it is telling you that the flexibility you seek is not there because you need more strength and coordination to accomplish the physical actions you have recently attempted (such as that new tennis serve technique) or else you will get hurt. In some cases, decreased flexibility is related to underlying injury or disease, such as intervertebral disk damage or joint arthritis. In these situations, tightness is the way your body warns you to protect yourself from additional injury.

PSI will not only warm you up, but will also help you figure out what your body is trying to tell you when your muscles are tight. *PSI* will inform you if you merely need more warming up, or if you really need to be careful because something is wrong with a part of your body.

Oftentimes, it can be very easy to confuse cause and effect in medical conditions. For example, it is commonly believed that tightness of the hamstring muscles causes back problems and is incorrectly thought to be resolved by stretching. However, hamstring tightness can actually be a sign that a back problem is already present. In other words, the back problem *causes* the hamstring tightness, and the hamstring tightness acts as a protective mechanism set up by the body to tell you to be careful so you won't do further damage to your back. *The hamstring tightness will disappear when the back problem has been solved.* Simply stretching away hamstring muscle tightness not only silences what your body is trying to tell you, but also removes the body's defense.

Most of the time, advocates of stretching talk about muscle stretching as though the muscle has been removed from the body and the exercise is to be done only on the muscle. Very little attention is paid to the joints in these discussions, except to describe the range of motion. But because joints rely on muscles for protection, increasing relaxed flexibility without increasing muscular control is potentially dangerous.

An example of such a serious injury is non-contact rupture of the anterior cruciate ligament (ACL). The ACL is an important ligament that connects the bones of the knee joint, providing stability to the knee during pivoting and stopping. Rupture of the ACL is a devastating injury for athletes and a tremendous cost nationally, estimated at 250,000 injuries per year costing at least $1.5 billion annually in healthcare costs. As it turns out, the hamstring muscles are well known in stretching circles for being tight in athletes who perform all sorts of running and jumping sports, as well as skiing and dancing. The hamstrings are also well known for their resistance to stretching. The viscoelasticity effects of stretching can wear off in a few minutes. As a result, specific stretches have been developed just to overcome tightness of the hamstrings to get them to elongate more than the body wants. But these stretches can cause a lot of damage by decreasing hamstring power and control, and allowing the knee to rotate too much when it is near full extension. Because the hamstrings protect the ACL by controlling knee extension and rotation, stretching causes the hamstring to lose this ability and puts the ACL at risk.

Fortunately, coaches and trainers have recently started to rethink their approach to warm up and conditioning. Instead of stretching to straighten the knee, they now emphasize warm ups that increase control of the bent knee, resulting in decreased numbers of ACL injuries in athletes, particularly female athletes, who have three to four times as much risk of ACL injury as their male counterparts.

But Stretching Feels So Good . . .

Don't worry! You will feel even better with *PSI*, without the risks and negative effects of stretching! *PSI* will help you to wake up, warm up, feel good, have more energy, and increase your flexibility. Warming up with *PSI* will prepare your body for whatever fitness or sport activity you choose to, and will clear you for maximal effort while warning you if you should be careful of any impending injuries. Plus, *PSI* can be done anytime and anywhere.

ABOUT PAIN

Pain is your body talking to you. What is your body saying? In order to improve communication about pain, health care professionals have developed systems to measure pain, such as facial expression charts or numeric systems. Unfortunately, one person's 8 may be another's 2. This makes giving instructions about pain and exercise notoriously difficult. As you warm up with *PSI*, your body will talk to you. If you have problems, *PSI* will help you to understand what your body is saying by using the techniques in the "Language of Pain" section in Chapter 6, "When You're Sore." All you have to do is test your body with *PSI*.

Testing Your Body When You're Sore

Tightness, soreness, and pain are all messages from your body. You can simply turn these messages off by stretching, or, you can run a "preflight check" during warm up with *PSI*. Sometimes warm up is all you need to feel good. Sometimes your body is telling you that you have been pushing it hard, but there is no problem. Sometimes you may be heading for a problem because of faulty technique or from overdoing a new exercise. If so, you may want to get some coaching and slow down a bit. Finally, pain could mean that you already have a problem and should stop what you are doing and get help before you get in trouble. Warming up with *PSI* will help you figure all this out: Can you perform as hard as you want? Do you need to be careful? How much can you do? When should you stop? Should you get help? From whom? If something is not quite right because of your exercise, sport, or dance, *PSI* will give you a good idea what is wrong with your body and what caused it. *PSI* and *Natural Flexibility* will help figure out what's to blame—inadequate flexibility, overuse or poor technique, or irritated or damaged tissues.

NATURAL FLEXIBILITY BODY MOVEMENTS

Chapter 3

Warm-up

Body
Movements

A TRULY GOOD warm up not only prepares and protects you, but should also warn you when your body is having trouble with the demands of your exercise, sport, or dance and then tell you what to do about it. The basic warm-up technique in this chapter does all these things. If you have pain, basic warm up will direct you to Chapter 6: When You're Sore or Chapter 7: Your Chiropractor in Your Pocket, to learn why and what to do about it.

Sometimes a new technique or recently increased level of training is more than your body can handle, and when this happens, increased tightness or soreness is your body's way of saying that you may be heading for trouble with an overuse injury or pulled muscle. On the other hand, not all soreness is reason for worry. So how do you sort out ordinary pain and stiffness from the warning signs of overuse or injury? The warm up you will learn next is specially designed to relieve ordinary stiffness, soreness, and pain. Not only will you feel better, but you you'll be able to figure out what to do if stiffness, soreness, or pain returns. (For exercises that can help you understand and treat these problems, see Chapter 6: When You're Sore).

ALWAYS WARM UP

The first part of this chapter goes into detail explaining the 'hows' and 'whys' of basic warm up. If you'd rather get right to it, and you have no unusual soreness, skip to page 43. If you have questions, you can always look back at the details later.

Your body needs time to increase flexibility and re-activate muscles, balance, and coordination. The more time you spend warming up, the more you maximize these gains. The basic warm up in this chapter covers all necessary territory without wasting your time. However, if you do find yourself pressed for time, you can do the "6-Minute Warm Up" at the end of this chapter, plus some of the warm ups for the areas of your body that you feel need more work. So you've got no excuse not to warm up!

The most straightforward warm up is simply going through the motions of the exercise, sport, or dance you are about to undertake but at a low level of effort. Be careful and don't get carried away; you're not supposed to be in a full-throttle competitive or performance mode. Make sure to cover all bases.

PSI for Warm Up

While some athletes and coaches may still think that isometric exercise means pushing as hard as you can against a wall or trying to lift a huge weight, there is actually no need to perform *PSI* at maximum effort. In fact, not only can *PSI* be performed within a range of precisely controlled efforts from very gentle to strenuous, but *PSI* can also be used at any joint position and in any direction you want. This means that if you have a problem with a certain part of your body, you can take it easy and modify the isometric exercise to exactly the level you need in order to avoid pain.

Improved flexibility is an important goal when warming up, and because flexibility is important at all points in your range of motion, *PSI* is the perfect tool for warming up. By warming up with *PSI*, you increase your flexibility at all the other places in your range of motion and can even assess your flexibility at places where you can't stretch. Warm up with *PSI* starts in the safe mid-range of motion. For every muscle group you activate with *PSI*, you also activate the antagonist muscles (the opposite muscle group that stabilizes the action). As your warm up progresses, *PSI* keeps you constantly informed so you never exceed your zone of control and can even expand your zone of control as you warm up. Most importantly, *PSI* tells you what you can and cannot safely do when you discover something is not quite right.

Spinal and Abdominal Warm Up

Always warm up your back, neck, and abdomen first. Neck, back and abdominal warm up is crucial for powerful use of the arms and legs. The following set of exercises will get you ready to go without the dangerous maneuvers of stretching. Remember, to improve flexibility naturally, you never force your body. After this warm up, ordinary neck and back stiffness should disappear. If you feel you are especially tight, or if you have neck or back problems, you should read Chapter 7: Your Chiropractor in Your Pocket before you continue.

SET UP: Lie down on the floor or mat. Lift your buttocks up and place your hands, palms down, underneath your buttocks so the fingers overlap comfortably. They should be positioned like this.

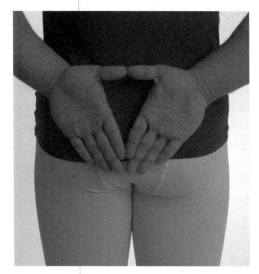

Set your buttocks back down on your hands. The purpose is to tilt your lower pelvis and hips forward slightly. The fingers need to be under the bony part of the sacrum and the fleshy part of the buttocks, not under your lower back. Adjust the position of your hands if necessary to support your pelvis comfortably and so that your hips move forward slightly as your lower back straightens out.

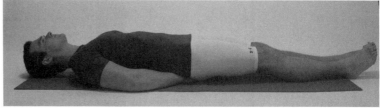

NATURAL FLEXIBILITY TECHNIQUE:
Spinal and Abdominal Activation

1. Gently lift your feet with your knees bent bringing your knees toward your chest. Don't force them. You will feel some tightness, but this should improve as you continue the exercise. Lift your head ½ inch from the floor and face the ceiling. Count to 30. Remember to breathe during the exercise. (Note: While this may seem like a kind of stretch, you are actually performing an isometric exercise for your abdominal and anterior spinal muscles in your neck and back, gently squeezing fluid out of your disks so they will become more flexible and less likely to be injured.) Put your legs and head all the way down to rest for 10 seconds, then repeat the exercise 2 more times.

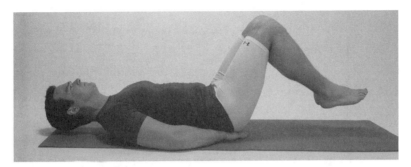

2. Assuming you are not sore, you are ready for more action. Straighten your legs out, but let your knees remain as bent as you need for comfort. Now, lift your head about ½ inch from the floor. Don't bend your neck to look at your feet.

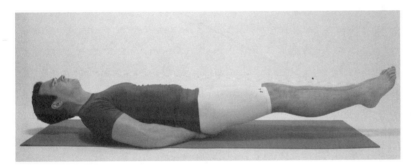

3. Keeping your hands under your pelvis, lift your legs as far as you feel comfortable. Let them down again to about one inch from the mat, and lift them up again. As you feel more limber, turn your head from right to left as much as you comfortably can. Breathe regularly with each leg lift.

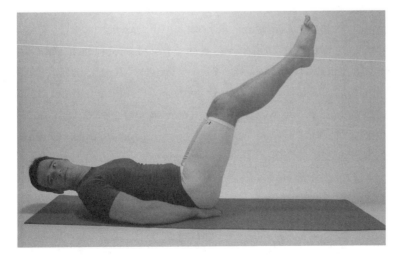

Besides improving the spinal activation you already began, this exercise improves your cardio-vascular adjustments for standing up. Repeat as many times as you are able without straining. A good warm up is 30 to 50 reps.

If you have pain during any of the above exercises, you should read Chapter 6: When You're Sore and Chapter 7: Your Chiropractor in Your Pocket to help figure out what is going on.

PSI TO WARM UP AND TEST YOUR UPPER BODY

You are now going to learn how to use *PSI* as a special exercise technique to warm up and test your upper body. Every exercise is done three times for a set. *PSI* is a progressive exercise, meaning that each time you repeat a particular exercise you use more effort, so how much effort you exert is up to you. But here are a few guidelines: The first exercise in a set is always very gentle. The second exercise is stronger. The third is even stronger, but never a maximum effort. *PSI* is also a sequential exercise, which means that you complete a group of similar exercises in one position and then start over again in a new position. *PSI* is also an isometric exercise, so you don't move at all during the exercise. The sequences are reciprocal because after you test and warm up one muscle group, you immediately test and warm up the opposite muscle group.

As we discussed earlier, *PSI* tests your body as it warms you up. These exercises are specifically designed to test every muscle group controlling your upper extremities, as well as the bones and joints. If you have pain during an exercise, **STOP!** Your body is telling you that something may be wrong. You must learn the Language of Pain. Go to Chapter 6: When You're Sore to find out what is going on and what to do about it.

The upper-body warm up can be done by itself, but you can always combine it with the lower-body warm up (below) to save time without cutting corners.

Upper body warm up involves 6 different exercise progressions, each named for the shoulder action being used: **IR** for **I**nternal **R**otation, **ER** for **E**xternal **R**otation, **FL** for **Fl**exion, **EX** for **Ex**tension, **AD** for **Ad**duction, and **AB** for **Ab**duction. To fully warm up the upper body, you should repeat all 6 exercise progressions in 5 different shoulder positions.

The 6 exercise progressions done at one shoulder position form a sequence. The first sequence we will demonstrate is called the Center Sequence, because the shoulder is in the center of its range of motion. Breathe normally during each of the exercises.

NATURAL FLEXIBILITY TECHNIQUE:

Center Sequence

Move your shoulders so you can place both your hands together comfortably in front of your body. Follow the instructions for each of the following 6 exercise progressions for the shoulder.

Center—IR

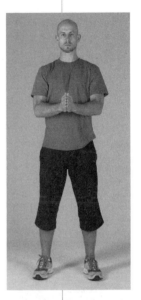

1a. Place the palms of your hands together in front of your body with your elbows bent at a right angle and, very gently, push your hands together for 10 seconds, like this. Breathe normally.

If you have no pain, progress to the next level of effort. Repeat this same exercise two more times, in the same position, just the way you did for the first exercise, and each time increase the effort by a comfortable amount. Remember to breathe normally.

Sports like tennis, golf, baseball, hockey, rowing and kayaking use this action frequently. The antagonist muscles and tendons that slow down and control this action are often the ones that get worn out first. You will start to warm them up now.

Center—ER

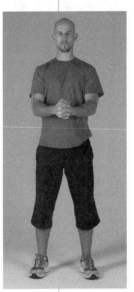

1b. Place your shoulders and arms in the same position that you did for the first exercise. Clasp your hands together and gently try to pull them apart for 10 seconds.

If you have no pain, progress to the next level of effort. Repeat this same exercise two more times, in the same position, just the way you did for the first exercise, and each time increase the effort by a comfortable amount. Remember to breathe normally.

The Center—IR and Center—ER exercises are a reciprocal pair. That is, the muscles you warm up perform opposite actions. Your body uses this reciprocal pair of muscles as a team. Almost all movements of your body rely on reciprocal pairs of muscles working as teams.

You are ready to warm up the next reciprocal pairs of muscles. The ways in which you exert the efforts are different, but the position of the shoulder and arms is the same.

If you have pain during the exercise, **STOP!** Go to Chapter 6: When You're Sore to find out what is going on and what to do about it.

Here is the next 10-second exercise pair in the center sequence:

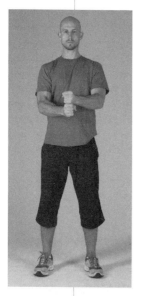

Center—FL

2a. Without changing position, make a fist with each hand and place the left fist on top of the right. Push your fists together for 10 seconds.

Repeat this same exercise two more times, in the same position, with increasing effort, just the way you did for the first exercise.

Center—EX

2b. Now switch positions of the hands. Without changing position, make a fist with each hand and place the right fist on top of the left. Push your fists together for 10 seconds.

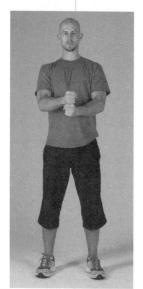

These two exercises are another reciprocal pair. Remember, each time you increase the effort during a set, only increase by a comfortable amount. It is always better to use less effort when in doubt. **Never** use maximum force for a warm up exercise.

Here is the last pair of exercises in the center sequence:

Center—AD

3a. Without changing the position of your shoulders, straighten your elbows out comfortably, but not all the way, and very gently, push your hands together and Count to 10, like this. Remember to breathe normally during every exercise.

Repeat this same exercise two more times, in the same position, with increasing effort, just the way you did for the first exercise.

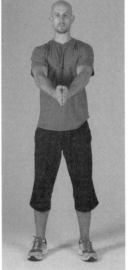

Center—AB

3b. Finally, without changing position at all, very gently try to pull your hands apart for 10 seconds.

Repeat this same exercise two more times, in the same position, with increasing effort, just the way you did for the first exercise.

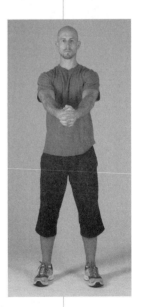

You have just completed the center sequence of the upper body warm up. Here it is all on one page:

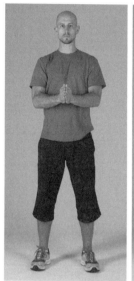 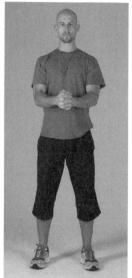

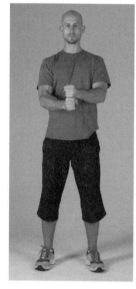 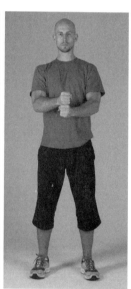

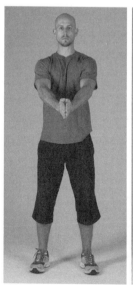 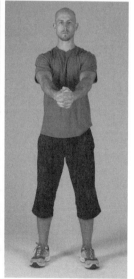

If you think about it, you will realize that the center sequence of basic warm up took only 3 minutes. Meanwhile, you started to test and warm up your shoulders, arms, elbows, forearms, wrists, and hands, along with all the muscles controlling them.

To fully test and warm up your upper body for vigorous sport or dance, you should do 4 more sequences, applying the same principles you used in the Center Sequence. Each sequence will be done in a different shoulder position. The sequences are named for the positions taken by the arms and shoulders. Each position should be at a comfortable limit of motion. Don't force the shoulders or other joints into uncomfortable positions. There is a Right-Down Sequence, a Left-Down Sequence, a Right-Up Sequence, and a Left-Up Sequence. Each will take 3 minutes, that is, about 15 minutes to fully warm up the upper extremities.

NATURAL FLEXIBILITY TECHNIQUE:
Right-Down Sequence

Move your shoulders so you can place both your hands together as far down and to the right of the front of your body as you comfortably can. For each of the above 6 exercises, **IR, ER, FL, EX, AD,** and **AB,** do sets of 3 progressive 10-second reps, as you did in the Center Sequence.

Here is the Right-Down Sequence on one page:

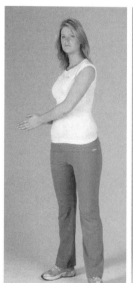
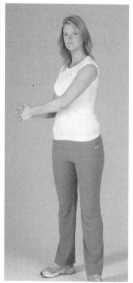
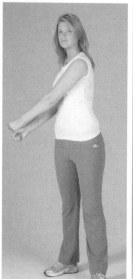
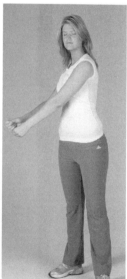
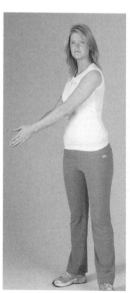
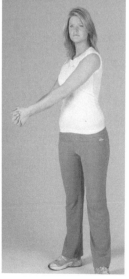

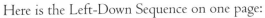

NATURAL FLEXIBILITY TECHNIQUE:

Left-Down Sequence

Move your shoulders so you can place both your hands together as far down and to the left of the front of your body as you comfortably can. For each of the above 6 exercises, **IR, ER, FL, EX, AD,** and **AB,** do sets of 3 progressive 10-second reps, as you did in the Center Sequence.

Here is the Left-Down Sequence on one page:

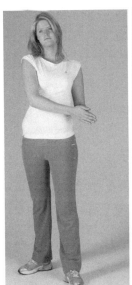
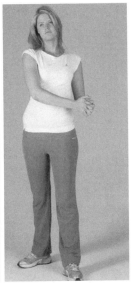
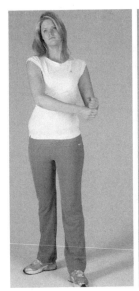
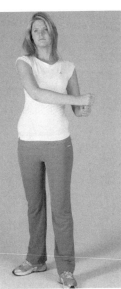
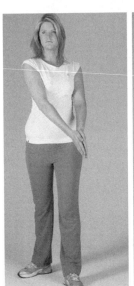
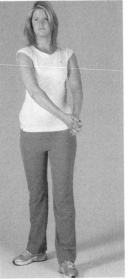

NATURAL FLEXIBILITY TECHNIQUE:

Right-Up Sequence

Move your shoulders so you can place both your hands together as far up and to the right of the front of your body as you comfortably can. For each of the above 6 exercises, **IR, ER, FL, EX, AD,** and **AB,** do sets of 3 progressive 10-second reps, as you did in the Center Sequence.

Here is the Right-Up Sequence on one page:

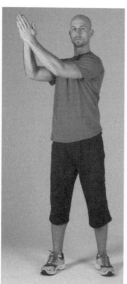
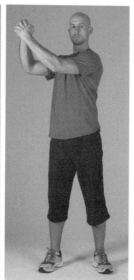
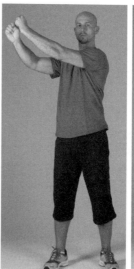
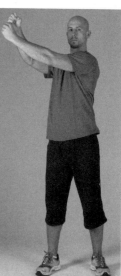
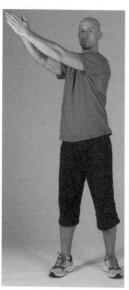
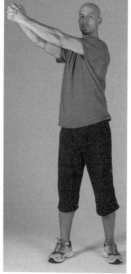

NATURAL FLEXIBILITY TECHNIQUE:

Left-Up Sequence

Move your shoulders so you can place both your hands together as far up and to the left of the front of your body as you comfortably can. For each of the above 6 exercises, **IR, ER, FL, EX, AD,** and **AB,** do sets of 3 progressive 10-second reps, as you did in the Center Sequence.

Here is the Left-Up Sequence on one page:

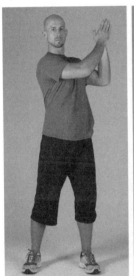
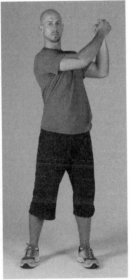

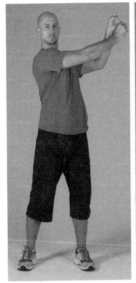
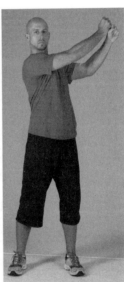

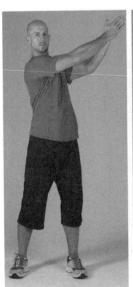
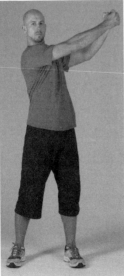

LOWER BODY WARM UP

Cardiovascular fitness relies on lower-body fitness and preparation. Running, cycling, skiing, skating, and dancing develop cardiovascular fitness primarily through the action of lower extremity muscles that are much larger and more powerful than those of the upper extremity. So a lower-body warm up should include preparation for cardiovascular fitness activities. It should likewise include an effort to develop good balance, which improves your sense of joint position and is the key to good footwork and optimum performance. Good balance prevents injuries more effectively than almost anything else. (Balance is the ability to hold yourself or move with control within a weight-bearing posture. Balance requires activation of the central nervous system as well as preparation of the musculoskeletal system for rapid reflexive adjustments.) Good balance relies on strength much more than is commonly appreciated. You cannot expect to have good balance if you have not developed the strength you need for an action.

If you have pain during an exercise, **STOP**! Consult Chapter 6: When You're Sore for help to figure out why and what to do next. Use your arms for balance, as you see fit. If you prefer, when you have become familiar with the lower body warm up, you can do basic upper body warm up at the same time.

SET UP: Effective lower body warm up relies on keeping your weight on the front of your foot with a bent knee. Let's look at two stages of shifting your weight to the front of your right foot.

In the easy stage, when you stand on your foot with your weight forward, your heel still takes some of the weight.

The harder stage is when you stand on the ball of your foot; your heel does not touch the ground.

When instructed to "Shift your weight to the front of your foot," you can use the easier stage of shifting your weight to the front of your foot as much as your need to, especially at the beginning. As you improve, you should use the harder stage as much as possible. So, let's get going.

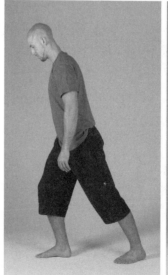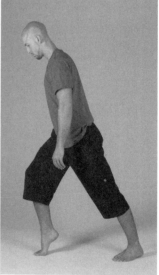

NATURAL FLEXIBILITY TECHNIQUE:
Side Balance Left Leg

1a. Stand comfortably with your legs spread at shoulder width. Shift your weight to the front of your feet. Keep your heels off the ground as much as you can. Shift your weight to your left knee and let it bend comfortably. Count to 10. Breathe normally.

2a. In the same position, shift more of your weight to your left knee so it bends a little more. Shift your weight to the front of your left foot as much as possible. Your right toes touch the floor to assist with balance. Count to 10. Breathe normally.

3a. Finally, in the same position, shift all of your weight to your left knee and the ball of your left foot. Lift your right foot off the ground about 1 inch. Count to 10.

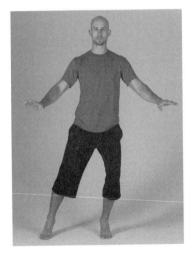
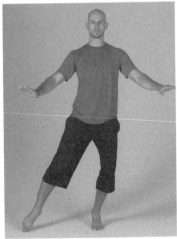
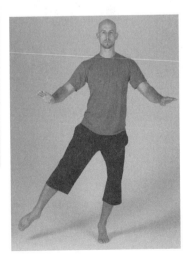

Now let's do the right side.

Side Balance Right Leg

1b. Stand comfortably with your legs spread at shoulder width. Shift your weight to the front of your feet. Keep your heels off the ground as much as you can. Shift your weight to your right knee and let it bend comfortably. Count to 10. Breathe normally.

3b. In the same position, shift more of your weight to your right knee so it bends a little more. Keep your weight to the front of your right foot as much as possible. Your left toes touch the floor to assist with balance. Count to 10. Breathe normally.

3b. Finally, in the same position, shift all of your weight to your right knee and the ball of your right foot. Lift your left foot off the ground about one inch. Count to 10. Breathe normally.

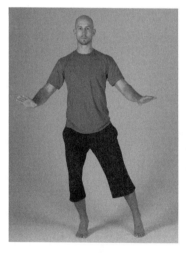
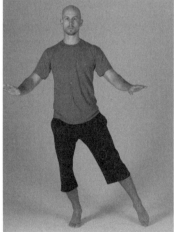
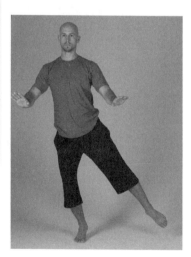

Here are two more common footwork positions where balance practice is usually needed.

Forward Balance Left Leg

1a. Step forward with your left foot and comfortably bend both knees. Shift your weight to the front of your left foot. Keep your heels off the ground as much as you can. Count to 10. Breathe normally.

2a. In the same position, shift more of your weight to your left knee so it bends a little more. Shift your weight to the front of your left foot as much as possible. Your right toes touch the floor to assist with balance. Count to 10. Breathe normally.

3a. Finally, in the same position, shift all of your weight to your left knee and foot. Lift your right foot off the ground about one inch. Count to 10. Breathe normally.

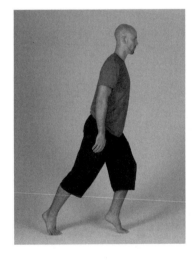
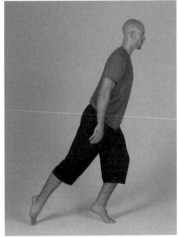
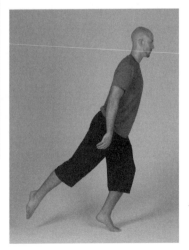

Now let's do the right side.

Forward Balance Right Leg

1b. Step forward with your right foot and comfortably bend both knees. Shift your weight to the front of your right foot. Keep your heels off the ground as much as you can. Count to 10. Breathe normally.

2b. In the same position, shift more of your weight to your right knee so it bends a little more. Shift your weight to the front of your right foot as much as possible. Your left toes touch the floor to assist with balance. Count to 10. Breathe normally.

3b. Finally, in the same position, shift all of your weight to your right knee and foot. Lift your left foot off the ground about one inch. Count to 10. Breathe normally.

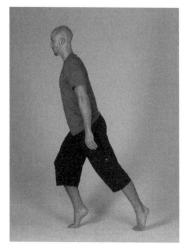
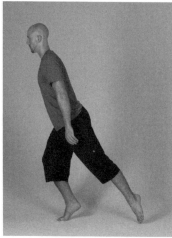
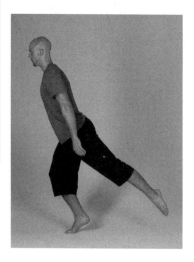

It is easy to imagine variations of these exercises for further balance improvement. For example, if you play tennis, you might practice right and left leg positions that are those you use as you hit a forehand or backhand.

CLOCK JACKS

Clock Jacks are a modification of traditional Jumping Jacks, which were popularized by Jack La Lanne, the Godfather of Fitness. Clock Jacks are aerobic exercises that build upon the balance, strength, and control you have just been working on. Clock Jacks use *plyometric principles*: with each jump, energy is stored in muscles and joints and used for the next jump. For optimum balance and injury prevention, this must occur in several different directions. Arms should be should be raised and lowered during the exercise and move opposite the feet to maintain balance.

SET UP: Pretend you are standing in the center of a clock face that has been placed on the ground. Twelve o'clock is straight ahead, three o'clock is on your right, six o'clock is behind you, and nine o'clock is on your left.

During each jump, bend your knees as much as you comfortably can and remain on the balls of your feet as much as possible. And, of course, you should breathe normally!

NATURAL FLEXIBILITY TECHNIQUE:
Clock Jacks

1. Starting with both feet in the center, jump so the left foot lands on nine o'clock and the right at three o'clock simultaneously.
2. Next, jump so both feet return to center, a traditional Jumping Jack sequence.
3. Next, the left foot jumps to six o'clock, the right foot to twelve o'clock.

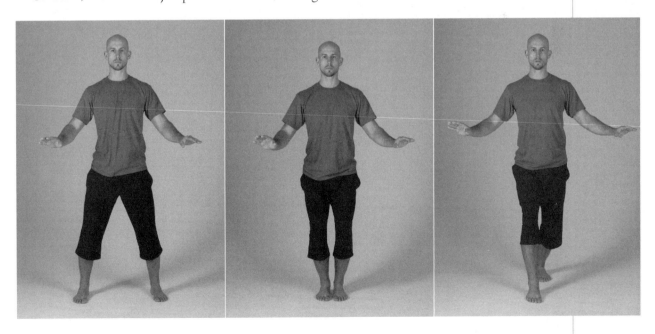

4. Then jump so both feet return to center again. At the next jump, the left foot goes to twelve o'clock and the right foot to six o'clock.

5. Return to center on the next jump, then jump so the left foot lands at 10 o'clock and the right foot at 4 o'clock simultaneously.

6. Then, jump so both feet return to center. Next, the left foot jumps to 8 o'clock, the right foot to 2 o'clock.

7. Finally, return to center on the next jump and repeat the sequence again.

Continue the Clock Jacks for at least 2 minutes.

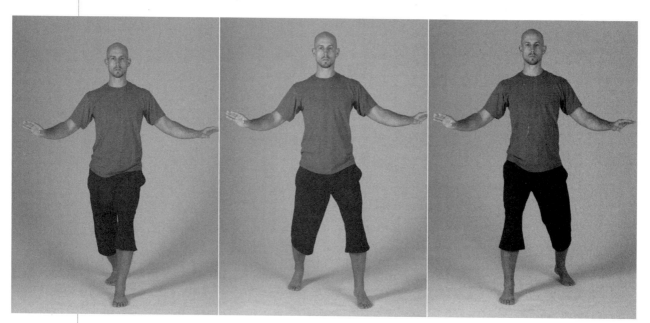

THE 6-MINUTE WARM UP

Stretching is no substitute for proper warm up. Here's a real-life example of why. It happened during the men's doubles final of our local tennis club. A crowd of spectators was already in attendance, waiting for the start of the match, and my son and I were on the court, fully warmed up and ready to go. Our opponents could be seen descending the long stairway from the parking lot. As they reached courtside, one of them dropped down to the ground and started to stretch both his ankles, saying, "I already tore one of my Achilles tendons, and my trainer says I need to do this before I play." We hit a bit, and then he started to serve. After a few points, my son returned a well-executed drop shot in front of the server, who raced in to retrieve it. As he did, we all heard a pop. He fell to the ground in agony, holding his previously uninjured ankle. He had ruptured his *other* Achilles tendon.

I can tell many stories about how stretching has let people down, but that one happened right in front of me. If you're running late or are otherwise limited on time, here's a safe, quick warm up that will not let you down. If you have pain as you warm up, or if you have an already-known problem, you should thoroughly test the sore area before you rely on this fast warm up.

NATURAL FLEXIBILITY TECHNIQUE:
Spine and Abdominals (about a minute and a half)

SET UP: Lie down on the floor or mat. Lift your buttocks up and place your hands underneath your buttocks, palms down, so the fingers overlap comfortably.

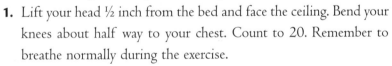

1. Lift your head ½ inch from the bed and face the ceiling. Bend your knees about half way to your chest. Count to 20. Remember to breathe normally during the exercise.

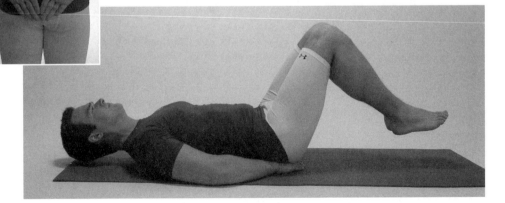

2. Straighten out your legs as much as you can, but let your knees remain as bent as you need for comfort. Lift your head about ½ inch from the floor.

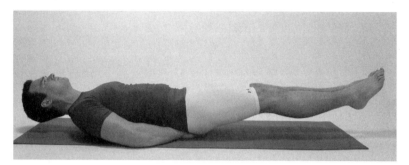

Keeping your hands under your pelvis, lift your legs as far as you feel comfortable. Let them down again to about 1 inch from the mat, and lift them up again. Don't bend your neck to look at your feet. With each rep, alternately turn your head slowly to the right or left. Repeat 30 times. Remember to breathe during the exercise.

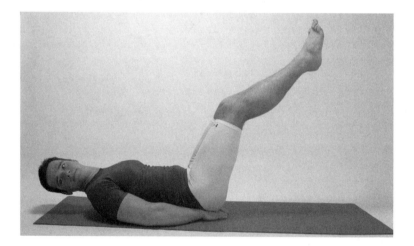

NATURAL FLEXIBILITY TECHNIQUE:

Upper Body (about 2 and a half minutes)

Upper body warm up involves 6 different exercises, each named for the shoulder action being used: **IR** for **I**nternal **R**otation, **ER** for **E**xternal **R**otation, **FL** for **FL**exion, **EX** for **EX**tension, **AD** for **Ad**duction, and **AB** for **Ab**duction. To fully warm up the upper body, you should repeat all 6 exercises in 5 different shoulder positions. The 6 exercise progressions done at one shoulder position form a sequence. The first sequence we will demonstrate is called the Center Sequence, because the shoulder is in the center of its range of motion. Breathe normally during each of the exercises.

CENTER SEQUENCE

Move your shoulders so you can place both your hands together comfortably in front of your body. Follow the instructions for each of the following 6 exercises for the shoulder.

Center—IR

1a. Place the palms of your hands together in front of your body with your elbows bent at a right angle and, with a moderate force, push your hands together for 5 seconds, like this. Breathe normally.

Center—ER

1b. Place your shoulders and elbows in the same position that you did for the first exercise. Clasp your hands together and, with a moderate force, try to pull them apart for 5 seconds. Breathe normally.

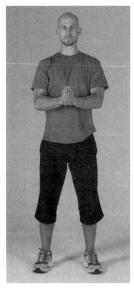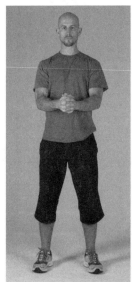

The Center—IR and Center—ER exercises are a reciprocal pair.

You are now ready to warm up the next reciprocal pairs of muscles. The ways in which you exert the efforts are different, but the position of the shoulders and arms is the same. Here is the next 5-second exercise pair in the center sequence:

Center—FL

2a. Without changing shoulder and elbow position, make a fist with each hand and place the left fist on top of the right. Push your fists together for 5 seconds with a moderate force.

Center—EX

2b. Now switch the hands' positions. Place the right fist on top of the left. Push your fists together with a moderate force for 5 seconds.

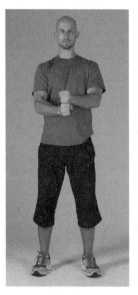 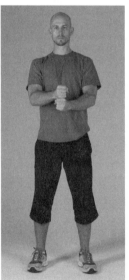

These two exercises are another reciprocal pair.

Here is the last pair of exercises in the Center Sequence:

Center—AD

3a. Without changing the position of your shoulders, straighten your elbows out comfortably, but not all the way, and with a moderate force, push your hands together and count to five, like this. Remember to breathe normally during every exercise.

Center—AB

3b. Finally, without changing position at all, with a moderate force, try to pull your hands apart for 5 seconds.

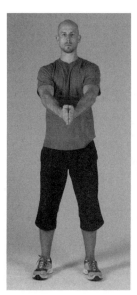 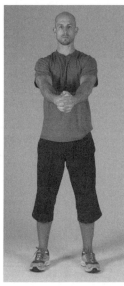

Here is the Center Sequence on one page:

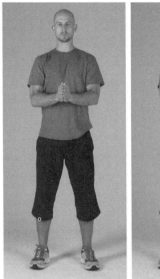 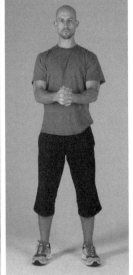

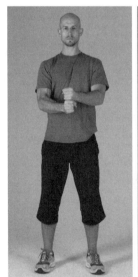 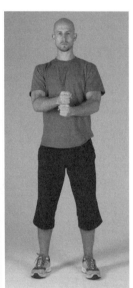

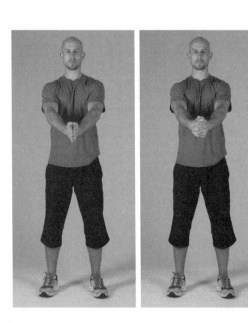

To complete the warm up for your upper body for vigorous sport or dance, you should do 4 more sequences, applying the same principles you used in the Center Sequence. Each sequence will be done in a different shoulder position. The sequences are named for the positions taken by the arms and shoulders. Each position should be at a comfortable limit of motion. Don't force the shoulders or other joints into uncomfortable positions. There is a Right-Down Sequence, a Left-Down Sequence, a Right-Up Sequence, and a Left-Up Sequence. Each will take 30 seconds. If you have more time, use it.

NATURAL FLEXIBILITY TECHNIQUE:

Right-Down Sequence

Move your shoulders so you can place both your hands together as far down and to the right of the front of your body as you comfortably can. For each of the above 6 exercises, **IR**, **ER**, **FL**, **EX**, **AD**, and **AB**, follow the instructions for the 5-second exercise, just as you did for the Center Sequence.

Here is the Right-Down Sequence on one page:

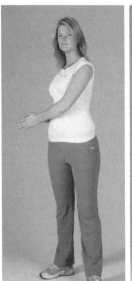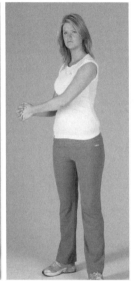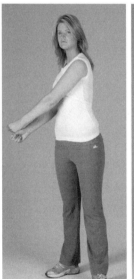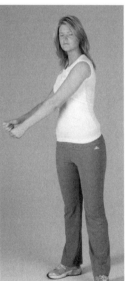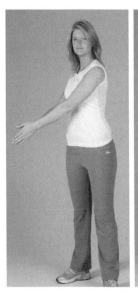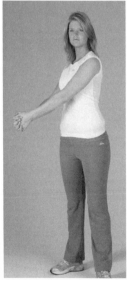

NATURAL FLEXIBILITY TECHNIQUE:

Left-Down Sequence

Move your shoulders so you can place both your hands together as far down and to the left of the front of your body as you comfortably can. For each of the above 6 exercises, **IR, ER, FL, EX, AD,** and **AB,** follow the instructions for the 5-second exercise, just as you did for the Center Sequence.

Here is the Left-Down Sequence on one page:

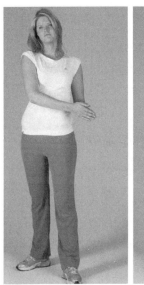
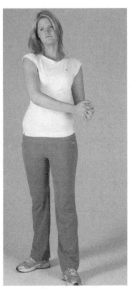
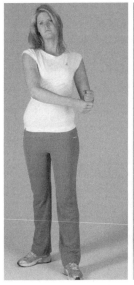
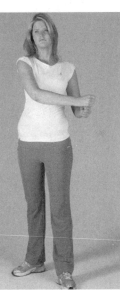
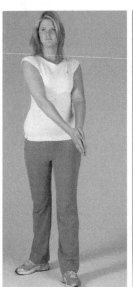
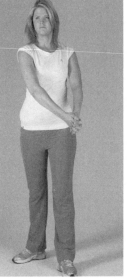

NATURAL FLEXIBILITY TECHNIQUE:

Right-Up Sequence

Move your shoulders so you can place both your hands together as far up and to the right of the front of your body as you comfortably can. For each of the above 6 exercises, **IR**, **ER**, **FL**, **EX**, **AD**, and **AB**, follow the instructions for the 5-second exercise, just as you did for the Center Sequence.

Here is the Right-Up Sequence on one page:

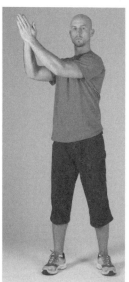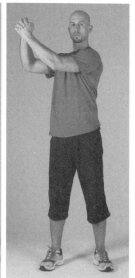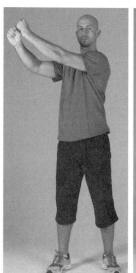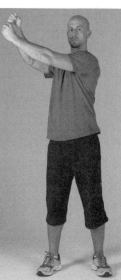

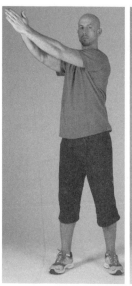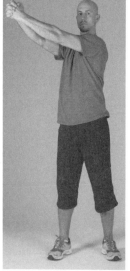

NATURAL FLEXIBILITY TECHNIQUE:

Left-Up Sequence

Move your shoulders so you can place both your hands together as far up and to the left of the front of your body as you comfortably can. For each of the above 6 exercises, **IR**, **ER**, **FL**, **EX**, **AD**, and **AB**, follow the instructions for the 5-second exercise, just as you did for the Center Sequence.

Here is the Left-Up Sequence on one page:

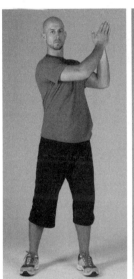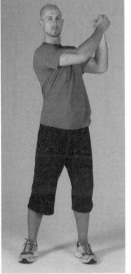

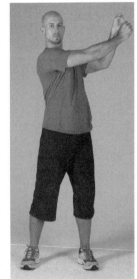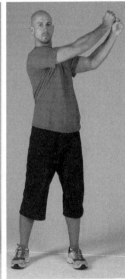

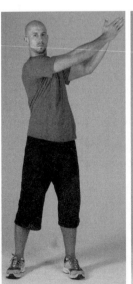

Clock Jacks for 2 minutes.

You should now be warmed up. If you had pain, and it is gone, you are ready for your workout, sport, or dance. If you still have pain after the warm up exercises, you will find out why and what to do about it in Chapter 6: When You're Sore.

Chapter 4

Wake-up
Body Movements

WAKING UP IS a daily opportunity that is commonly underappreciated. You have the choice each time you wake up to become fully aware of your body, yourself, and your world. Balance, poise, grace, and bearing follow in this focused awareness. As you lie on your back in bed after you awaken, your spine is relaxed and unstressed. Wake-up exercises should highlight and activate this effortless, individual posture you wake up with and teach you how to bring it with you all day. All you need to do is activate the miraculous mind-body endowments that you usually take for granted and often ignore. Then, just for a moment, pause long enough to remember how truly good you feel as the day begins. If you are reluctant to trade a few minutes of sleep for a refreshed, renewed start of the day, you should think twice. Why get out of bed tired? Try these exercises just once, in the morning. That's all you'll need to be convinced. After that, you'll never get out of bed tired again. For those in a real hurry, and in good shape, look at the 5-minute wake up at the end of the chapter.

MAKE THE MOST OF WAKING UP

You are now going to learn wake up exercises that are based on scientific medical studies, but you may also recognize principles of Pilates, martial arts, dance, and gymnastics. These exercises will literally open your eyes. You won't have to sweat. They are so simple that they only take a few minutes. For starters, you should know about the three components of wake-up exercises:

1. Arm and leg *PSI* activates the autonomic nervous system that opens the eyelids, modulates blood pressure and heart activity, and redistributes the circulation to permit sitting and standing.
2. Spinal *PSI* magnifies the activation of arm and leg *PSI* and prepares for trunk stabilization and extremity action. Spinal *PSI* is essential to prevent and alleviate neck and low back pain.
3. Put it all together to combine muscular action, postural control, balance, and attitude.

You may vary these exercises. For example, if you increase the force of the exercises, you will wake up faster. If you decrease the force of the exercises, and repeat them, you will slow, and intensify the process of waking up. As you become familiar with them, you may want to focus on some and eliminate others.

UPPER-BODY AND AUTONOMIC WAKE-UP EXERCISES

SET UP: These exercises can be done without removing the covers or your pillow. You don't even have to open your eyes. Remember to breathe during each exercise. Since these exercises are designed to be done while you are still very sleepy, you should familiarize yourself with the first few of them the night before. After you do the first few exercises, you will be awake enough so you can refer to this book again, if it is close at hand. Soon, you will do them automatically when you first awaken from sleep.

NATURAL FLEXIBILITY TECHNIQUE:
Autonomic Activation

1. Lie flat in bed, arms at your sides, palms down. Slowly, very slowly, without any force at all, with your elbows almost straight and your arms still at your sides, lift your arms

so your elbows and hands just barely come off the bed, no more than an inch or two, and spread your fingers gently. Count to ten and put your hands back on the bed.

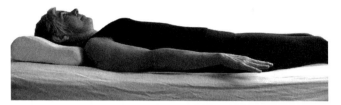

2. With the same small amount of force that you used to lift them up, push the palms of your hands against the bed. Keep your elbows straight and arms at your sides. Count to ten.

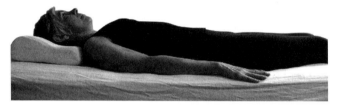

If you wish, repeat the above two exercises one or two more times. Each time, use slightly more force. Again, remember to breathe during each exercise. Don't hold your breath.

3. With your hands still at your sides, turn your arms so your palms face upward. Slowly, but not tightly, close your fists. Gently lift your arms so your elbows and hands are about one inch from the bed and hold them for a count of 10, gently tightening your fists as you do it. Return your hands and arms to the bed.

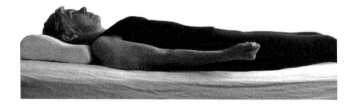

4. Open up your fingers. Push against the bed with the back of your hands using the same gentle force you used to lift up your hands.

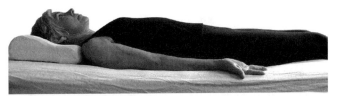

If you wish, repeat the above two exercises one or two more times. Each time, use slightly more force. Breathe during the exercises.

5. With your elbows straight, bring your hands together in front of your body and clasp your hands together. Keeping your elbows straight and keeping your hands clasped together, try to pull your hands apart. Use the same gentle force you originally used to lift up your hands. Count to 10.

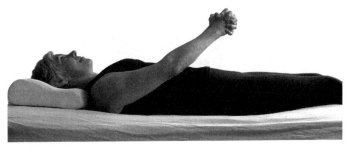

6. Unclasp your hands, spread your fingers apart, place your fingertips together and push them gently. Count to 10.

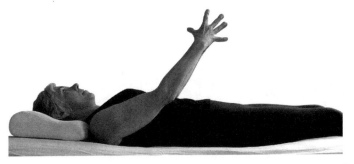

If you wish, repeat the above two exercises one or two more times. Each time, use slightly more force. Remember to breathe normally.

7. Bend your elbows. Clasp your hands together again. Try to pull your hands apart for 10 seconds.

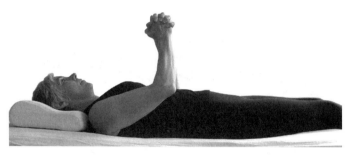

8. Then, with your elbows still bent, unclasp your hands, spread your fingers apart, place your fingertips together, and push them together gently. Count to 10.

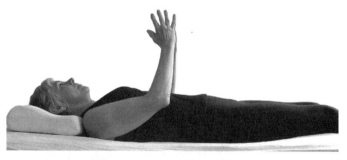

If you wish, repeat the above two exercises one or two more times. Each time, use slightly more force. Remember your breathing.

9. Again, with your elbows bent, make a fist with each hand. Place your left fist on top of the right. Tighten your fists and gently push them together. Count to 10.

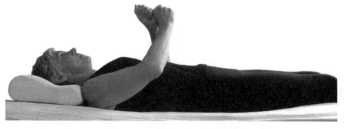

If you wish, repeat the above two exercises one or two more times. Each time, use slightly more force. As before, breathe during each exercise and don't hold your breath. Then, reverse the position of your fists, keeping your elbows bent and repeat the above exercises.

NATURAL FLEXIBILITY TECHNIQUE:

Upper Extremity Flexibility

1. Remove the blanket from the top part of your body. Lift up both arms, spread your fingers, and point your fingertips toward the ceiling. As you do so, lift up the backs of your shoulders so that your arms move toward the ceiling. Count to 10.

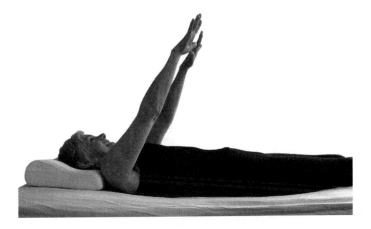

2. Make a fist, but not too tightly. Bend your elbows and lower your shoulders and gently push your shoulders back into the bed. Count to 10.

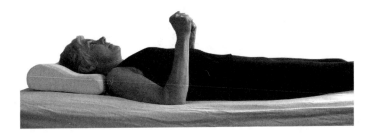

3. If you wish, repeat the above two exercises one or two more times. Each time, use slightly more force, and remember to breathe naturally.

SPINAL, ABDOMINAL,
AND LOWER BODY WAKE-UP EXERCISES

SET UP: If you have not already done so, remove your pillow. Let your head settle back comfortably. With your hands at your sides, bend your knees and place your feet on the bed. You may wish to remove the blanket completely for this exercise. Lift up your buttocks and place your hands underneath your buttocks, palms down, so the fingers overlap comfortably.

Set your buttocks back down on your hands. The purpose is to tilt your lower pelvis and hips slightly forward. Hence, the fingers need to be under the bony part of the sacrum and the fleshy part of the buttocks rather than under your lower back. Remember—don't place your hands under your back.

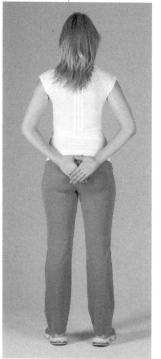

Adjust the position of your hands if necessary to support your pelvis comfortably and so that your hips move forward slightly as your lower back straightens out. Bend your knees comfortably. This is the starting position.

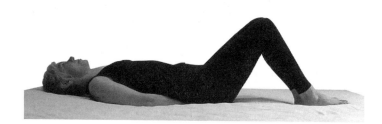

NATURAL FLEXIBILITY TECHNIQUE:
Isometric Core Activation

1. Gently lift your feet an inch or two from the bed with your knees bent. Lift your head ½ inch from the bed and face the ceiling. Count to 30. Remember to breathe during the exercise.

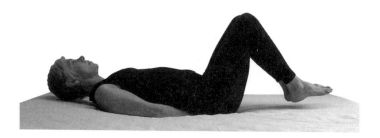

2. Straighten your knees a bit. Keep looking at the ceiling. Once again, lift your head about ½ inch and your feet a few inches. Because your knees are straighter, slightly more effort will be required. Count to 30. Remember to breathe properly.

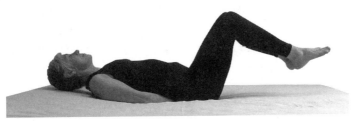

3. Remove your hands from behind your buttocks and place them at your side. Keep looking at the ceiling. Keep both knees straight during this exercise. Lift your right leg a few inches from the bed and hold it for a count of 30.

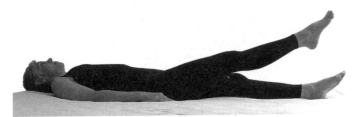

4. Place your right leg back on the bed. Now lift your left leg a few inches from the bed and hold it for a count of 30.

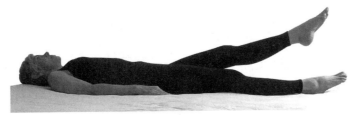

5. Alternate a few more times with each leg as much as you wish. Remember to breathe properly. This exercise works the quadriceps and iliopsoas muscles of the leg you lift and the hamstrings of the opposite leg. It is probably the safest hamstring exercise there is.

NATURAL FLEXIBILITY TECHNIQUE:

Dynamic Core Activation

You are now ready to be more dynamic. We'll be repeating the wake up movements with slightly more intensity.

6. Straighten out your legs more, but let your knees remain as bent as you need for comfort. Place your hands under your pelvis as before. Lift your legs as far as feels comfortable. It is important to face the ceiling as you lift your head about ½ inch from the bed. Don't bend your neck to look at your feet.

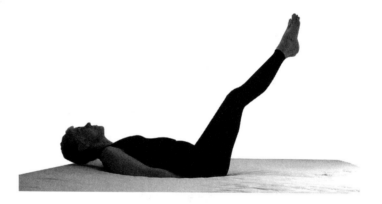

Let them down again to about 1 inch from the bed, and lift them up again. Repeat as many times as you are able without strain. While 30 is a good number of repetitions, you may only be able to do 5 or less when you are first starting.

Remove your hands from behind your buttocks and place them at your side. Now it's time to get out of bed.

RISE AND SHINE

You will now learn how to take the effortless, natural posture you already have in bed and bring it with you when you sit and stand. Focus upon and remember the light, energized feeling you have when you take these first steps of the day. You will automatically "refresh" your posture anytime you recall this feeling later on. You will have a totally different way to renew your body, your mood, and your posture simply by recalling how you felt in those first few moments when you woke up. Now you will link your freshly activated autonomic nervous system with the physical readiness of *PSI*.

As we proceed, always remember that your head is the key to keeping the natural relaxed position you already have in bed.

SET UP: Normally, when you awaken and lie in bed without a pillow looking straight ahead, your head is already lined up with your spine and you are using no effort whatsoever. With your knees bent, you could be sitting on the edge of the bed with the same effortless posture.

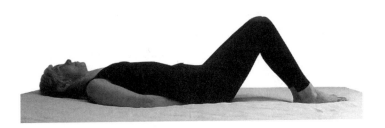

So, when you sit at the edge of the bed, your posture should be about the same as when you were lying down with your knees bent. It is the same when you're standing up. There shouldn't be much difference in your posture from when you were lying down. The relationship of your head and spine remain the same.

Next you will learn how to take this effortless posture you have while lying down and bring it with you for the rest of the day. All you need to do is balance your body. But first, you have to get out of bed with gymnastic attitude.

NATURAL FLEXIBILITY TECHNIQUE:
Rise and Shine

As you did the leg lifting exercises, you probably realized that the momentum of your legs could actually lift your upper body off the bed if you moved your legs fast enough. This is the basis for a well-known acrobatic maneuver called the *kip-up*. If you are too forceful, you actually can kip-up out of bed unintentionally and land on the floor, so be careful! You are not going to kip-up out of bed yet! Practice using your legs to bring you upright. Don't use much effort, and don't try to go all the way up. Get a feeling for how much force you need to exert in order to sit up. At the same time, make sure you preserve the relationship between your head and the rest of your upper body. Try to use the momentum of your legs to bring yourself part way up, like this. Don't sit all the way up yet. It's fine if you fall back down right away.

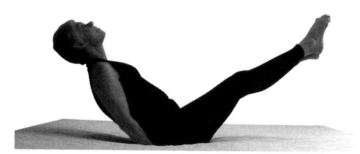

It should look like a Pilates exercise. We are especially interested in the position of your head related to your upper body and the alignment of your neck and back. We want the position to be the same that you had when lying down. Don't make any undue effort to keep your knees straight, or to point your toes or fingers. But don't let your neck, shoulders, or back slouch from that original position. Think of your body as a see-saw with its center somewhere near your belly button. Focus on keeping your head and spine in the same relationship you had when you were lying down. Use the momentum of your legs to rock up and down. Then, lie back down again, paying attention to your head and shoulders. Did they hit the bed at the same time as your back? If not, try it again until they do. You should master this before you progress to the next step. When you sit up the way we want, you will be balanced and light. You will be looking straight ahead, head slightly tilted up.

Practice until you have a good feeling for how much effort it takes to sit up this way. Make certain you are bringing your head up with the same relation to your upper body and spine that you had when you were lying down.

Next, you are going to arrange yourself in your bed so that, when your legs carry your head and upper body forward and up, you will end up sitting on the edge of the bed. Once you figure out where to sit, you should lie back, bring your legs up, and place your fingertips as a localizer at the edge of the bed. You do not want to end up too close to the edge of the bed or you will sail out of bed and onto the floor.

You should now be ready to sit up using the technique you just practiced. You should be able to judge how much force you need to exert with your legs to sit up all the way. You have activated your core stabilizers, your autonomic nervous system, and your extremities, so your eyes should be open. This way of getting up will give you the jumpstart on an attitude you can use for the rest of the day.

Now, with your arms in front of you, use the power of your leg lift to bring your upper body into a sitting position on the edge of the bed. Bend your knees as you do so, and plan to place your feet so only the balls touch the floor. Make sure your head stays in the same relationship to your upper body that it has when you are lying down. Your shoulders should be relaxed and your feet should be slightly behind your knees. Keep looking straight ahead. Slowly, as you count to 30, lean forward at your hips and gradually put your weight onto the balls of your feet. Don't curve your back or neck as you lean forward—keep them the way they were as you first sat up. If you do this properly, you will feel the quadriceps muscles in the front part of your thighs automatically begin to tighten in preparation for making you stand up. (Note: If you have trouble with your feet, you may not be able to stay on the balls of your feet).

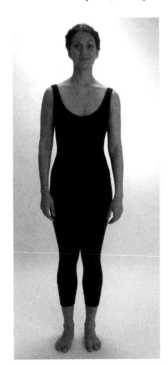

Keep your hands out in front of you for balance. If you have problems with your knees, you may need some help from your hands at this point. Keep your head in relation to your upper body as before. If you want, pick a spot on the wall ahead of you to use as a focal point . As you lean further forward, your buttocks will come off the bed and your quadriceps will tighten more to automatically stand you up. Let them.

You should now be standing. It is the beginning of a new day.

CLOCK STEPPING

Studies have shown that having good balance is one of the most important ways to prevent injury. You may still slip on that ice or trip over that shoe, but your body will react and save you from serious harm. A few moments of balancing exercise using Clock Stepping will not only get you ready for the day, but will provide accumulating benefits over time. Now is also the time to focus on that refreshed, energized feeling you have as you start the day.

Clock Stepping promotes the coordinated action of the energized body and mind for balance and controlled power. Clock Stepping relies on activated spine and abdominal muscles to stabilize the trunk and head and permit the effective use of the arms and legs. It is a one-legged strengthening and balance exercise that is essential to reducing the risk of a fall and/or injury.

SET UP: The arches of your feet, the ligaments and muscles that control your toes and ankles, and all the other supporting structures of your legs and spine become stronger as you practice your balance. It commonly takes at least 6 weeks to begin to have the strength needed for proper balance. Don't rush, or you will get sore.

Remember the natural position of your head with respect to your spine as you do these exercises. It is important to link the two feelings together: posture and balance. You have activated all the systems you need to do this, so it should be easy and effortless.

NATURAL FLEXIBILITY TECHNIQUE:

Developing Balance

You should be standing with your weight on both feet in a comfortable position. Place your arms in a natural position, ready to help with your balance. This is an example of a starting position.

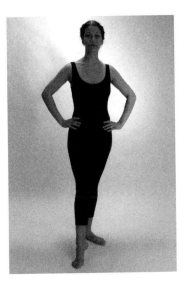

1. Shift your weight slowly to the right side and onto your right foot, bending your right knee slightly. Rise up on your left foot.

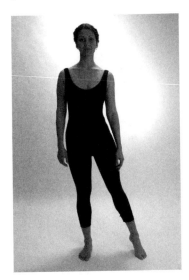

2. Shift your weight completely to the right side, touching the floor only with the toes of your left foot if you need to for balance. Lift your arms away from your sides as needed. Maintain your head and upper body position. Don't look at your feet. Count to 10.

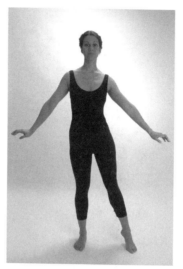

3. Shift your weight slowly to the front of your left foot as you bend your left knee and place the ball of your right foot on the floor. Maintain your head and upper body position. Count to 10.

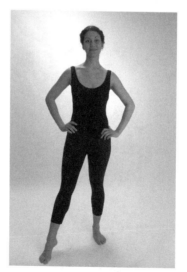

Shift your weight completely to the left side. Lift your right foot and place it further to your right, touching the floor only with the toes of your right foot if you need to for balance. Lift your arms away from your sides as needed for balance. Maintain your head and upper body position. Don't look at your feet. Count to 10.

You can now slowly shift your weight back and forth between the two feet, alternating the two positions.

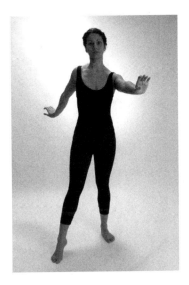

NATURAL FLEXIBILITY TECHNIQUE:
Clock Stepping

If you have more time when you wake up, here is a great way to develop wonderful balance. This method can be used any time of the day to revitalize your posture, as well as for a warm up before athletics or dance. You won't need to practice all the exercises all the time. Try different ones each time.

Now imagine that each foot is placed on a clock face: the right foot at 3 o'clock, the left foot at 9 o'clock. You can alternately shift your weight the same way as you just did for balance practice.

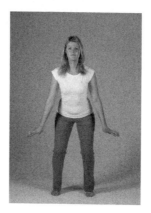

Be sure to keep your knees bent.

1. Let's make things more interesting. For the easier level, shift your weight completely to the right and further forward onto the right foot. At the same time, take all your weight off your left foot, using only the toes touching the floor. Balance on your right foot this way as you count to 30.

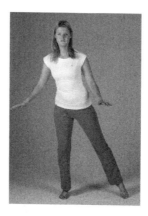

2. Now, for the harder level, with all your weight on the right foot, keeping your right knee slightly bent, rise up onto the ball of your right foot. At the same time, lift your left foot up. Do not touch the floor with your left foot unless you must for balance. Hold this position for 30 seconds, or for as long as you can.

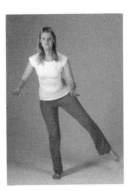

3. Now you are going to balance on your left foot at 9 o'clock. Shift your weight completely to your left foot, bending your left knee. Repeat the exercise at both levels of difficulty.

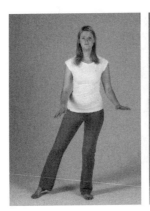 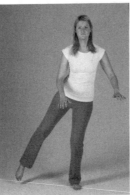

4. Next, place your right foot at 1 o'clock and your left foot at 7 o'clock. Shift your weight onto your right foot. Repeat the same 2 levels of exercise with your weight completely on your right foot. Maintain your head and upper body position and keep your right knee bent.

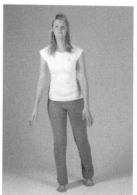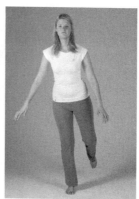

5. Then, shift your weight to your left foot. Repeat the 2 exercises.

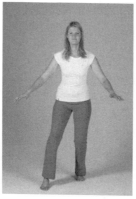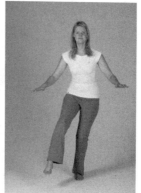

6. Next, place your right foot at 5 o'clock and your left foot at 11 o'clock. Shift your weight to your right foot. Repeat the same 2 levels of exercise.

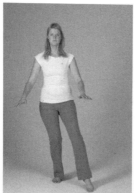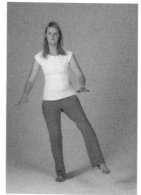

7. Then, shift your weight to your left foot. Repeat the 2 exercise levels.

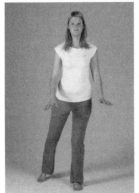 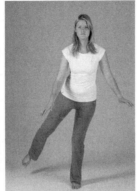

8. Next, place your right foot at 6 o'clock, your left foot at 12 o'clock. Shift your weight to your right foot. Repeat the 2 exercise levels.

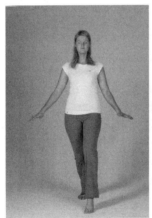 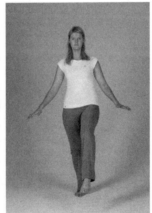

9. Then, shift your weight to your left foot and repeat the same 2 exercise levels.

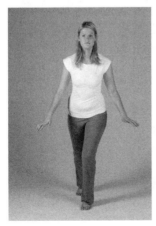 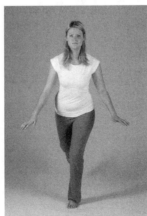

10. Finally, place your right foot at 12 o'clock, and your left foot at 6 o'clock. Shift your weight to your right foot and repeat the 2 levels of exercise. Be sure to maintain your head and upper body position and keep your right knee bent.

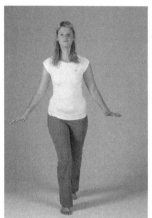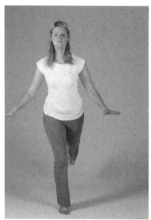

11. Shift your weight to your left foot and repeat the 2 levels of exercise.

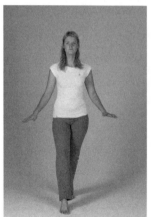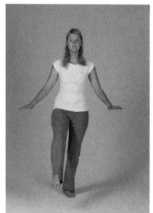

THE 5-MINUTE WAKE UP

This sequence up will activate your whole body with special focus on your back, neck, and abdomen. If you already have neck or back pain, I recommend taking a look at Chapter 7: Your Chiropractor in Your Pocket. While the 5-minute wake up won't enable you to capture all the great energy available to you as you awaken, I realize that sometimes you have no choice but to opt for a shorter wake up routine. So for those times when you only have a few minutes, use this routine to make the most of your wake up.

Isometric Core Activation

SET UP: As you lie on your back, face up, lift up your buttocks and place your hands underneath your buttocks, palms down, so the fingers overlap comfortably, like this:

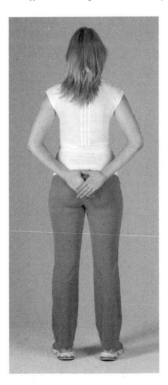

Set your buttocks back down on your hands.

NATURAL FLEXIBILITY TECHNIQUE:

1. Gently lift your feet an inch or two from the bed with your knees bent. Lift your head ½ inch from the bed and face the ceiling. Count to 30. Remember to breathe during the exercise.

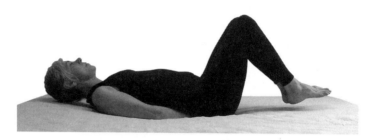

2. Straighten your knees as far as you feel comfortable. There is no need to straighten them all the way. Keep looking at the ceiling. Once again, lift your head about ½ inch and your feet a few inches. Because your knees are straighter, slightly more effort will be required. Count to 30. Remember to breathe properly.

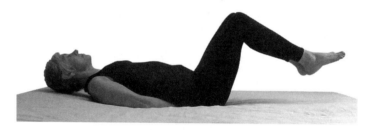

Dynamic Core Activation

SET UP: If you have room, move to the edge of the bed for a 1-minute set of leg lifts. Otherwise, do them where you are.

NATURAL FLEXIBILITY TECHNIQUE

1. Straighten out your legs more, but let your knees remain as bent as you need for comfort. It is important to face the ceiling as you lift your head about ½ inch from the bed. Keeping your hands under your pelvis, lift your legs as far as you feel comfortable. Let them down again to about 1 inch from the bed, and without letting them set down all the way, lift them up again. Repeat as many times as you are able in a minute. While

30 reps is a good number, you may only be able to do 5 or less when you are first starting.

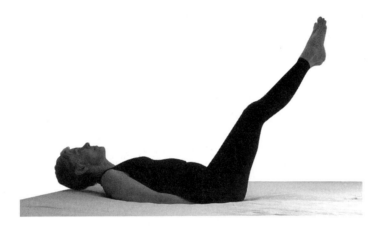

Taking Your Effortless Posture With You All Day

SET UP: Now it's time to sit up. You are going to take the natural, effortless postural alignment of your head and spine as you are lying down into the upright position. Then, you will learn to keep it by improving your balance. If you are already at the edge of the bed and have room, sit up by using the momentum of your legs at the end of the last leg lift, like this.

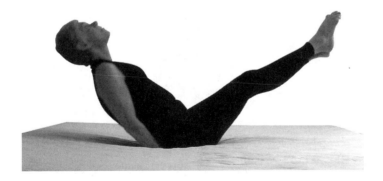

If you are not already at the edge of the bed, move there now and do one final leg lift, with a little more thrust, to sit up. This is a gymnastic maneuver and I want you to have a gymnastic attitude. The momentum of your legs should have carry you upright without any need to bend your neck or back. Your shoulders should be relaxed and your feet should be slightly behind your knees. Keep looking straight ahead. Balance your head on your spine. Balance, not effort, should

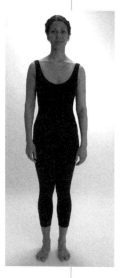

maintain the relationship of your head, shoulders, and spine. Then, slowly, lean forward *at your hips* and gradually put your weight onto the balls of your feet. *Don't curve* your back or neck as you lean forward—balance them the way they were as you first sat up. Feel the quadriceps muscles in the front part of your thighs automatically begin to tighten to automatically stand you up. Let them.

1. Shift your weight slowly to the right side and forward on right foot, bending your right knee slightly. Rise up on your left foot.

2. Shift your weight completely to the right side. Lift your left foot and place it further to your left, touching the floor only with the toes of your left foot if you need to for balance. Lift your arms away from your sides as needed for balance. Maintain your head and upper body position. Don't look at your feet. Count to 10.

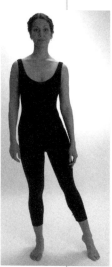

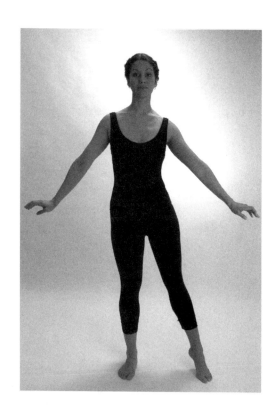

3. Shift your weight slowly to the front of your left foot as you bend your left knee and place the ball of your right foot on the floor. Maintain your head and upper body position. Count to 10.

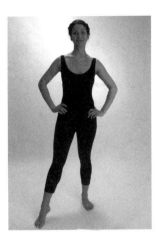

Shift your weight completely to the left side. Lift your right foot and place it further to your right, touching the floor only with the toes of your right foot if you need to for balance. Lift your arms away from your sides as needed for balance. Maintain your head and upper body position. Don't look at your feet. Count to 10.

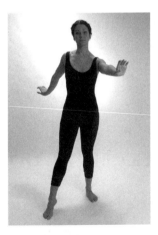

You can now slowly shift your weight back forth between the two feet, alternating the two positions. Stay on the balls of your feet as much as possible.

Good Morning!

Chapter 5

Advanced
Natural
Flexibility

THE AMATEUR ATHLETE can be sure that a basic warm up with *PSI* guarantees the best possible preparation for an enjoyable sports activity without the risks and performance impairments of stretching. The professional athlete, gymnast, skater, and dancer require no less than maximum flexibility for peak performance.

DYNAMIC FLEXIBILITY: ULTIMATE *PSI*

I am now going to show you exactly how to achieve all the flexibility benefits you wanted to have from stretching without the risks and performance drawbacks of stretching. This technique is called Ultimate *PSI* and is done at the maximum flexibility position. The maximum flexibility position lies at the end of the range of motion of any joint after it is warmed up, provided you move the joint into this position under its own control. Ultimate *PSI* is not a mere catchword here. It refers to the furthest your body wants you to go. Listen to your body as you develop your flexibility. Joint stability requires the combined action of agonist and antagonist muscles.

If you pull, push, or otherwise artificially force your joint using some other means than its own muscle power (like you do with a relaxed stretch) you may go beyond your maximum flexibility position and out of your zone of control.

You must first understand the basic principles underlying Ultimate *PSI* and stretching because, even though they look so much alike, they are very different.

A static stretch is done by relaxing a muscle and then pulling on it while it is relaxed so that it lengthens as much as can be comfortably tolerated. Ultimate *PSI*, however, is a series of progressive isometric exercises done at the maximum flexibility position. During Ultimate *PSI*, the muscle is always contracting; the muscle *does not* relax.

In Section I we discussed the science underlying flexibility and learned that isometric exercise increases flexibility through viscoelasticity effects just as much as stretching does. When you compare the negative training effects and risks of stretching with the performance-enhancement and injury-reduction benefits of isometrics, you realize that isometric exercise is the only smart way to increase your flexibility.

NATURAL FLEXIBILITY TECHNIQUE

Start gently. Over weeks of practice, you should be able to increase the effort you use during the third stage of Ultimate *PSI*. As you do, you will increase the strength and dynamic flexibility of the most important muscles in your shoulder and arm to prevent overuse injuries in pitching, golf, and tennis. Precisely controlled contractions of these same muscles are crucial to powerful energy storage and release during the wind up, backswing, and follow-through. Muscles shorten and elongate during these maneuvers, but they do not relax.

The key to Ultimate *PSI* is <u>not</u> to relax the muscles during the exercise. I would like you to start with a few simple isometric warm-up exercises to illustrate this very important point.

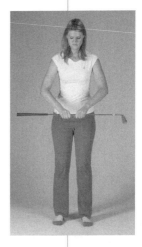

1. Grip a golf club firmly and pull on it with both hands using a gentle force for 10 seconds, like this. The force should be directed so that, if the golf club could get longer, it would.

2. Repeat this exercise two more times, each time with gradually increasing force.

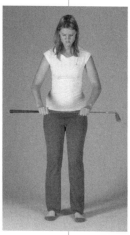
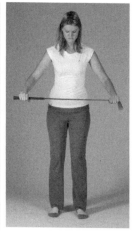

3. Move your hands apart a bit and pull again for 10 seconds.

4. Repeat this exercise two more times, each time with gradually increasing force.

5. Move your hands farther apart and pull again for 10 seconds.

6. Repeat this exercise two more times, each time with gradually increasing force.

Ultimate *PSI* Technique

So far, you have performed a series of isometric warm-up exercises in slightly different shoulder positions. Ultimate *PSI* should be done in a similar way. However, because we want to be especially careful that you are not tempted to pull your right arm into each new position using your left hand, I am going to ask you to let go of the club with the left hand temporarily at the end of each exercise. *Your right arm should move into each new position under its own power and control.* So, you must let go of the club with your left hand for each position change. You will never pull with your left hand unless you are also pulling with your right hand, exactly as you did with the simple exercises above that you just finished.

NATURAL FLEXIBILITY TECHNIQUE:

First Stage Ultimate PSI: Right Shoulder, Elbow, Arm

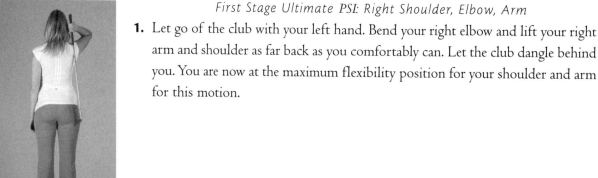

1. Let go of the club with your left hand. Bend your right elbow and lift your right arm and shoulder as far back as you comfortably can. Let the club dangle behind you. You are now at the maximum flexibility position for your shoulder and arm for this motion.

2. Now take it, but *do not pull it*, with your left hand. Now, just as you did a moment ago, pull on the club with both arms for 45 seconds using a moderate, gradually increasing effort, so neither hand moves.

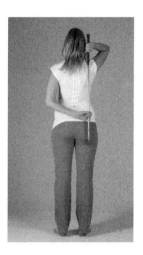

Second Stage Ultimate PSI: Right Shoulder, Elbow, Arm

3. Let go of the club with the left hand to make sure you are not pulling. Using only the power of the muscles of your right shoulder and arm, move the right shoulder back as far as you can. You should be able to move a little further than you did before because you have just increased the viscoelasticity of the muscles, tendons, and joints that you used to perform the isometric exercise. Therefore, your maximum flexibility position will have increased.

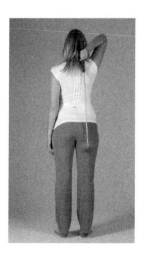

4. Grab the club again with your left hand but do *not* pull yet. Get both arms set, then pull with both hands and arms for 45 seconds the same way you have been doing, so that neither hand moves. Do not pull with the left arm and hand until the right arm and hand are also pulling. Do not pull harder with the left arm and hand than you can with the right arm and hand. If you feel very comfortable with your effort, you may gradually increase the effort equally with both arms over the 45-second period, but no motion should occur. You should feel more tension develop in the shoulder. Never exert so much effort that you lose control.

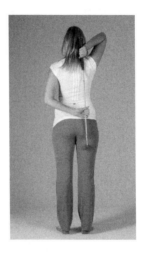

Third Stage Ultimate PSI: Right Shoulder, Elbow, Arm

5. Stop pulling with both hands. Let go of the club with the left hand to make sure you are not pulling. Using *only the power of the muscles of your right shoulder and arm*, move your right shoulder and arm back as far as you can once more. You should find that your maximum flexibility position has increased as you did the exercises.

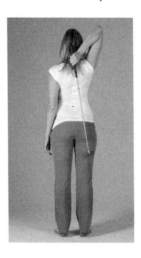

6. Grab the club again with your left hand, but do *not* pull yet. Get both arms set, then pull with both hands and arms for 45 seconds the same way you have been doing, so that neither hand moves. Do not pull with the left arm and hand until the right arm and hand are also pulling. Do not pull harder with the left arm and hand than you can with the right arm and hand.

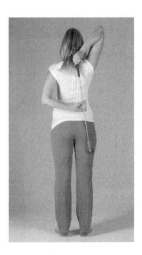

If you feel very comfortable with your effort, you may gradually increase the effort even more, provided you pull equally with both arms, so no motion occurs. You should feel more tension develop in the shoulder. Never exert so much effort that you lose control.

If you now test your shoulder's range of motion for a tennis serve or windup for a pitch, or in preparation for a wrestling match, you will find that it compares with what you would get from having stretched it for the same amount of time. But you already know that your improved flexibility is much better than stretching because you have activated all your muscles. Weeks from now, the regular training you get from your natural flexibility program with Ultimate *PSI* will not only give you increased range of motion, you will also have earned greater strength and control—and better protection from injury.

CONVERTING COMMON STRETCHES TO ULTIMATE *PSI*

It's time to convert some other common sports stretches into Ultimate *PSI*. Whatever muscles you were going to stretch just need to be activated during the exercise instead of relaxed. You can think of it as a resisted stretch as long as you don't get confused and actually start to stretch the muscles. It's very simple—the key is not to relax. And there should be no movement during the exercise. Also, to change position between exercises, always move your body naturally, under its own control. Never stretch or pull your body into a position. And always warm up first. Ultimate *PSI* is *not* a warm-up technique. Ultimate *PSI* is a dynamic flexibility technique.

In order to convert any stretch into an Ultimate PSI, you simply resist the stretch so no motion occurs. Each rep should be about 45 seconds. After each rep, use your own muscle power, not some outside force, to bring the joint into an increased flexibility position. Do not relax.

Use increasing, moderate force with each rep, but never use maximum force until you have become thoroughly familiar with your state of flexibility. Usually, this takes about six weeks. After each rep, your maximum flexibility position should increase as your flexibility increases. Over time, you will increase both your maximum flexibility and your strength and control in this position.

Always warm up first. Ultimate *PSI* is a not a warm-up technique. After basic warm up, approach the maximum flexibility position by first performing a series of progressive sequential isometric exercises, *PSI*, at comfortable mid-range positions in the range of motion (similar to what you did with the golf club the first few times you pulled on it). Each time you finish an isometric sequence, you move closer to the maximum flexibility position and repeat the sequence. It is very important that the muscles of the joint you are working do the moving from one sequence position to the next, so you can listen to your body, and allow your muscles to tell you how much flexibility you truly have. Never pull the joint with your other arm or leg, like you do with a stretch. Never force it into the next position using your body weight or gravity or some other means, as is commonly done with stretching. If you think you can buy a little more "flexibility" by pulling the right arm with your left you are buying false flexibility. You want flexibility with harmony and control. You want dynamic flexibility—flexibility with power. Similarly, if you work with a partner, never let your partner move your body into any position or overpower your effort. Your partner simply resists what you do, no more.

The muscles that you are going to work during Ultimate *PSI* control the motion of the joint in the maximum flexibility position. These muscles protect the joint from going beyond its safe limits. They also retrieve the energy stored in a back swing or wind up for peak performance.

Now, we are going to take a series of common stretches and convert them to Ultimate *PSI* using the principles we just went over. Remember to warm up first. For each Ultimate *PSI*, instead of relaxing as you would if you had stretched, you are going to perform three 45-second isometric exercises starting gently, with gradually increasing effort. Use the power of the muscles of the joint being worked to move closer to the flexibility limit position for the next exercise. Don't cheat by using some outside force to move the joint closer to the limit. In some cases, we demonstrate the use of a partner. The partner should not move your body, but should only resist your effort after you have positioned your body all by yourself. At the end of each 45-second isometric, your flexibility will have increased.

So, for each of the following exercises, move your body into its maximum flexibility position under its own power. Don't force it. Perform the isometric exercise at the maximum flexibility position for 45 seconds, using a gradually increasing force, WITHOUT MOVING. Rest 30 seconds. Repeat the exercise 2 more times, with 30 second rests between reps. Your flexibility should increase after each rep, so move into your new maximum flexibility position each time before you start the next rep. We have exaggerated the progression to demonstrate the idea that flexibility increases as you perform the exercise.

Tennis serve (left handed): Try to straighten left elbow, but resist with right hand.

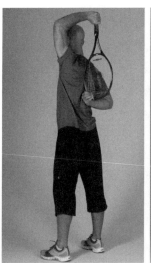 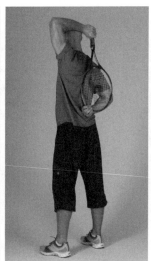 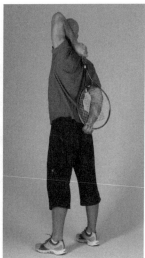

For the backhand (left handed): Try to hit the backhand, but resist with the other hand.

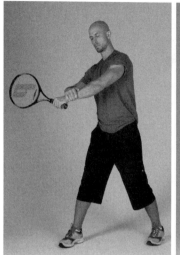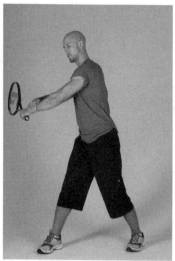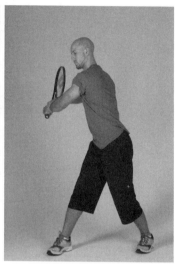

Take the club back as much as you feel comfortable. Your partner will take the club, but NOT PULL. You will try to swing the club, but your partner will prevent it from moving.

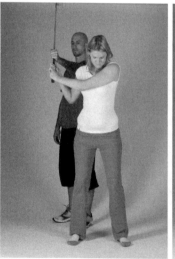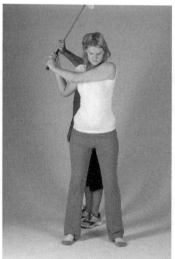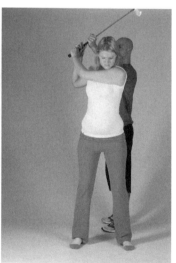

To work the antagonists and improve your follow through, bring the club into the full follow-through position. Your partner will take the club, but NOT PULL. You will try to swing the club the wrong way (opposite direction of follow through), but your partner will prevent it from moving.

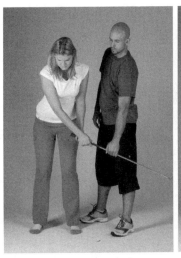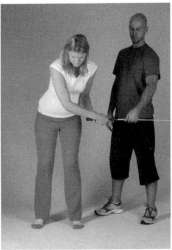

For basic hip flexibility a couple of *PSI* warm ups: Lift one or both hips about 45 degrees and hold for 45 seconds. Rest 30 seconds and bend the hip as much as comfortable. Holding that position, push against your thigh for 45 seconds. Rest 30 seconds, then bend the right hip as much as comfortable and repeat one or more times.

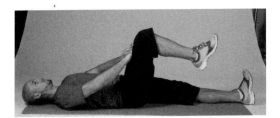

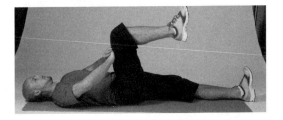

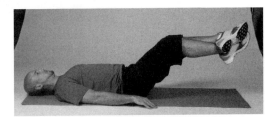

Or, alternatively: Start with hip bent just a little. Holding that position, push against your thigh for 45 seconds. Rest 30 seconds, then bend the right hip about 45 degrees and repeat. The last rep is with the hip bent up as much as you can.

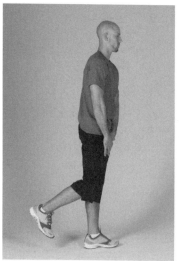 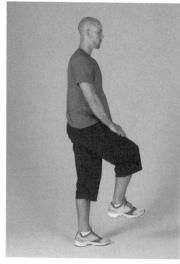 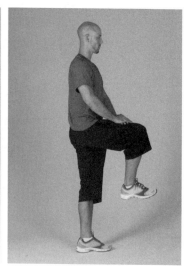

Squat with both hips bent about 30 degrees and hold for 45 seconds. Rest 30 seconds and bend the hips to about 45 degrees, and hold for 45 seconds. Rest 30 seconds, then bend the hips as much as comfortable and repeat one or more times.

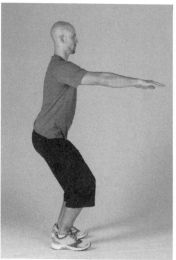 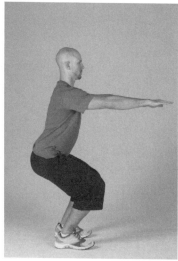 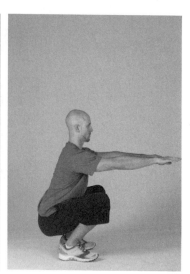

Sit with both hips bent, feet together, knees comfortably apart. With opposite hands, push against both knees and hold for 45 seconds. Rest 30 seconds, then spread the knees as much as comfortable and repeat two more times.

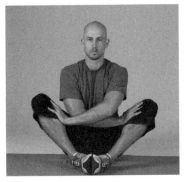 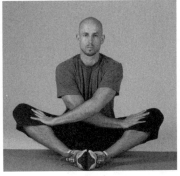 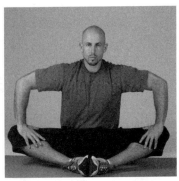

Starting now where you just left off, switch hands and try to pull your knees together and hold for 45 seconds. Rest 30 seconds, then bring the knees as close together as comfortable and repeat two more times.

The following may look like quadriceps stretches but they are not! They should be undertaken very gently at first. Be sure you warm up.

With the hip and knee comfortably bent, grab your ankle, BUT DO NOT PULL. Gently try to straighten your knee, but resist with your hand. Hold for 45 seconds. Rest 30 seconds, then straighten the hip and bend the knee as much as comfortable. Repeat two more times. Remember not to stretch.

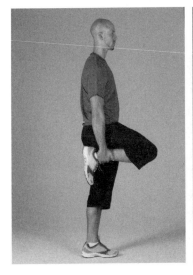 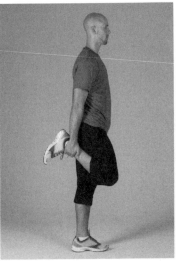 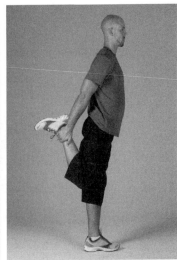

The most gentle hamstring exercise, great after pulls. Pay attention: this is a RIGHT hamstring exercise. In the first stage, you lift the LEFT leg. Note also that the hands are not touching the floor. If this first stage is too hard, bend the LEFT knee and put the hands down on the floor, so less effort is required. Until you actually try this exercise for yourself, you may not believe it works your hamstring. Gently try to straighten your hip, but resist with your hand. Hold for 45 seconds. Rest 30 seconds, then bend the RIGHT hip as much as comfortable, with the knee bent midway. Rest 30 seconds. Repeat with the hip bent more and the knee straighter, depending on how you feel.

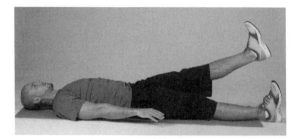

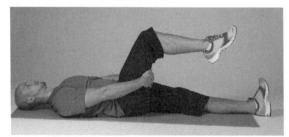

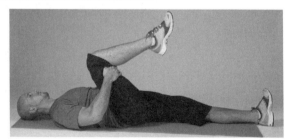

Again, the next exercise will look a lot like a stretch, so be careful! This is a RIGHT Achilles isometric progression. The right calf muscle should be activated and pushing during the entire exercise. DO NOT RELAX.

Stand with your weight on the right leg and rise onto the ball of your right foot. Hold for 45 seconds. Rest 30 seconds. Then, lift your right leg off the floor, bend your right ankle a little more (use the right leg muscles to do it), and replace the right foot further backwards, touching the floor only with the ball of your right foot, as you increase the amount of weight you put on the right foot. Rest 30 seconds and repeat. Note: never set your right heel down and always keep the right calf muscles pushing your right foot against the floor.

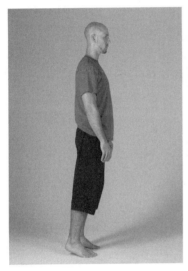
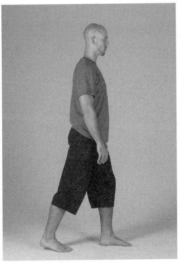
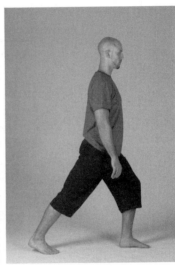

SECTION III:

ASSESSING

AND

ALLEVIATING

PAIN

Chapter 6

When

You're Sore

WHEN YOU'RE SORE, how do you know how much you can do in your sport or dance without getting hurt? For example, you may have shoulder pain and wonder if you can play tennis. When you try an overhead throwing motion, like a serving motion, your shoulder hurts. If you stretch it, it still hurts and feels tight. Can you play?

People often stretch when they're sore. Sometimes they do it to feel better, even though stretching can impair performance and cause injury. Sometimes they think they are going to prevent injury, but this is wrong. With no option, athletes and dancers often go ahead with their sport or dance even though they still feel sore.

HOW TO TEST YOUR BODY WHEN YOU'RE SORE

Not all pain or soreness is reason to avoid your sport or exercise. If you expect to use your body to stay fit, have fun, or earn a living, you must expect to have some wear-and-tear stiffness, soreness, and yes, even pain. So, first of all, any worthwhile test must tell you the difference between ordinary soreness and stiffness, and the abnormal pain of a developing problem. It should warn you if you are having a serious problem and help you to understand why. The test should also tell you what you can and cannot safely do. Most importantly, the test should tell you what to do about it.

I am going to take you through a simple testing process that can help figure all this out, but first of all, you must remember that pain can be a sign of a serious medical problem. If your pain is accompanied by other signs or symptoms, such as fever, weight loss, weakness, numbness, swelling, rash, or any other abnormality, you must see your doctor. If your pain is severe, getting worse, or spreading, you must see your doctor. If your pain lasts longer than a few days, keeps you awake at night, or prevents you from doing your normal activities, you must see your doctor.

Most people are completely in the dark about why they're sore. During my 30-year career in orthopaedic surgery, I have seen many athletes and dancers with avoidable injuries who had ignored their bodies' warning symptoms. In my experience, much of the time, athletes and dancers fail to recognize that they do have a developing problem, so the problem gets worse. I am going to try to help you to do better. I want to teach you early warning signs that something is wrong so it can be addressed before it gets worse. On the other hand, if you already think you have a problem and you were going to consult your doctor about it, do it! Consult your doctor! Never use these test exercises to decide not to see your doctor. I am going to try to give you some idea about what may be going on, but these tests cannot diagnose your medical problems.

The testing process is similar for most sore joints, muscles, tendons, and bones in your body, but at the beginning, we will focus on the *right* shoulder as an example. After we go through the process for the right shoulder, I will show you exactly how to test any other sore spot. You must be careful as you test yourself. Always start out with a very gentle effort. Never exert a maximum effort. Use good judgment. If you are unusually sore, don't take any risks. Consult your doctor. Any exercise, even a gentle test, presents some risk that you will make matters worse. The progressive tests that you will now learn are designed to warn you if you have a problem with your body before you start your sport or exercise, so they should be safer for you than doing the sport or exercise without knowing about the problem. If you are not sure about how safe it is to test a sore part of your body, ask your doctor first.

You already started this testing process if you came here from Chapter 3: Warm-up Body Movements. We are going to continue the testing process using *PSI*. Once you understand the principles of this chapter, you can include testing as part of your regular warm up without any extra fuss. If you have a chronic shoulder problem, for example, you will quickly become familiar with how to test it and warm up at the same time. I will show you how to test any sore muscle or joint, but there is no need to test areas of your body that are not sore; basic warm up will do. But if you discover a new painful area, you will want to have *Natural Flexibility* close at hand.

Actions, Positions, Results

Here is the first key idea: Tightness, soreness, or pain that is due to decreased flexibility, and only to decreased flexibility, should go away as you increase your flexibility during the testing. So, the ideal test exercise should increase your flexibility as you do the test. Sometimes your flexibility needs more work than others, so the test exercise should take that into account as well. Any pain that remains after you increase your flexibility is due to some kind of developing problem.

The second key idea is this: A developing problem with a **muscle or its tendon** will cause pain whenever you perform the **action** of that particular muscle. A problem with the **surface of your joint,** or with **a ligament or other tissue in the joint**, will cause pain whenever you put the joint in the **position** that irritates or catches that particular tissue. Some problems, like rotator cuff tears, can be combinations of problems of action and irritation. Therefore, to fully test a region of your body that is sore, the test exercises you use must cover all the important muscle **actions** as well as test the joint in different **positions.** Furthermore, the test exercise must not catch or damage already sore tissues, so you must not move while you do the test. You also must be able to do the exercises as gently as needed to prevent additional irritation. Finally, you must be able to start with the joint in a safe mid-position and only attempt more difficult positions after you begin to increase your flexibility.

The beauty of progressive sequential isometric exercise is that it does all that.

TESTING YOUR BODY WITH *PSI*

Testing the sore places in your body with *PSI* is easy. *PSI* is a progressive exercise technique, meaning that for each test exercise set, there will be three levels of effort: The first exercise in a set is always very gentle, for example, the equivalent to holding a weight of only I to 5 pounds. The second exercise is stronger, perhaps 3 to 10 pounds of force. The third is even stronger, perhaps 10 to 15 pounds of force or more, but never a maximum effort. You must be the judge of how much force to apply with each level of effort. Remember, these exercises are supposed to test and warm up your body as they increase your flexibility. They are not intended to make you stronger while you do them! The set of test exercises done at all 3 levels of effort make up a test exercise progression for that action.

To test all the actions of the right shoulder, for example, you perform 6 test exercise progressions, each named for the shoulder action being tested: **IR** for **I**nternal **R**otation, **ER** for **E**xternal **R**otation, **FL** for **FL**exion, **EX** for **EX**tension, **AD** for **AD**duction, and **AB** for **AB**duction.

You test all 6 actions without changing the position of your shoulder. Then, you move your shoulder to 4 other positions and repeat the same 6 actions for each position.

The 6 shoulder actions done at one shoulder position form a sequence. The first sequence we will demonstrate is called the Center Sequence, because the shoulder is in the center of its range of motion, the safest and most stable position.

The Language of Pain

As you do a test exercise, your body answers you with a test result, using the Language of Pain. There are 5 possible test results for every test exercise:

Result 1: You have no pain during the exercise.
Result 2: The pain disappears during the exercise.
Result 3: The pain is less during the exercise, but it is still there.
Result 4: The pain is unchanged during the exercise.
Result 5: The pain is worse during the exercise.

We will now start to test your body with *PSI* using the right shoulder as an example. Every time you get a new result from a test exercise, you will interpret the result using the Language of Pain for the level of effort you used.

FIRST LEVEL 10-SECOND TEST EXERCISE
FOR YOUR SHOULDER

Center—IR

Move your shoulders so you can place both your hands comfortably in front of your body. Place the palms of your hands together with your elbows bent at a right angle and, very gently, push your hands together and Count to 10, like this. Breathe normally.

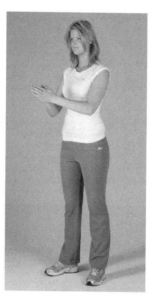

You have just used *PSI* to test your shoulder. What did you figure out?

Interpreting Your First Level Test Result
Using the Language of Pain

For a moment, we'll look at all five possible test results. When the time comes to really test a sore part of your body, you will look only at *your* result.

Result 1: You have no pain during the exercise. This is a good sign. Your body is telling you that it is not experiencing any problem from doing this particular exercise. You will be able to progress to the second level of effort for this 10-second test exercise.

Result 2: The pain disappears during the exercise. You have pain at first during the test exercise, but the pain disappears during the exercise.

It is likely that the pain was related to lack of flexibility. *PSI* increased your flexibility during the test and the pain went away. You will be able to progress to the second level of effort for this 10-second test exercise.

Result 3: The pain is less during the exercise, but it is still there. You have pain during the test exercise, the pain is less intense as you do the exercise, but the pain is still there when you finish the exercise.

It is likely that the pain is related to lack of flexibility and you have not increased your flexibility enough. You may also have some underlying tissue irritation or weakness. To figure this out, you need to do this exercise for a longer time to increase your flexibility. You must repeat the same test exercise at the first level of effort for an additional 45 seconds.

Then, look at your new test result for the first level, just as you did after the 10-second test exercise.

Note: Your next result will direct you back here if the pain is again less, but some pain still remains after you finish the 45-second test exercise. If so, rest 30 seconds and repeat the same 45-second test exercise, in the same position, at the same first level of effort that you just used. Look once more at your new test result for the first level.

If you are directed here a third time, rest for another 30 seconds and do the 45-second test exercise for a third and final time at the first level of effort.

PSI increases your flexibility each time you do a 45-second flexibility exercise, up to a total of three exercises at the same level of effort. No benefit comes from doing a 45-second flexibility exercise more than three times at the same level of effort. Pain due to lack of flexibility should go away as you increase your flexibility. If you still have pain after three 45-second exercises, it means there might be something else causing the pain in addition to lack of flexibility. Nevertheless, *since your pain has been decreasing during the exercises,* a slightly greater effort may be all that is needed to increase your flexibility enough to get rid of the pain. Progress to the second level of effort for this 10-second test exercise.

Result 4: The pain is unchanged during the exercise. You have pain during the test exercise, and the pain is the same when you finish the exercise.

It is possible that the pain is related to lack of flexibility and you have not increased your flexibility enough. You may also have tissue damage or weakness. To figure this out, you must repeat the same test exercise for an additional 45 seconds. Then, look once more at your new test result for the first level.

Note: If the pain remains the same during the 45-second test exercise, you will be directed back here. If so, rest 30 seconds and repeat the same 45-second test exercise, in the same position, at the same first level of effort that you just used. Look once more at your new test result for the first level.

If you are directed here a third time, rest for another 30 seconds and do the 45-second test exercise for a third and final time at the same first level of effort.

If the pain is the same after three repetitions of the 45-second test exercises at the same level of effort, **STOP!** Something may be wrong. You have completed this test exercise progression. Your test result is 4. Move on to the next first-level test exercise progression.

Result 5: The pain gets worse during the exercise. You have pain as you do the test exercise and the pain gets worse during the exercise.

STOP! This is a sign of tissue damage or weakness. Your body is telling you to protect these tissues. In the Language of Pain, increasing pain means your body is telling you to stop this particular action and to avoid it until damaged tissues heal and are strong enough to perform the action. So **STOP!** Find out what is wrong. You must avoid this action. If you cannot avoid this action during your exercise, don't exercise. If you feel you cannot participate in your sport or dance if you have to avoid this particular action, don't participate! You may get hurt. You should consult a sports medicine physician, or orthopaedist before you do this particular exercise. You have completed this test exercise progression. Your test result is 5. If you wish, you can move on to the next first-level test exercise progression.

SECOND LEVEL 10-SECOND TEST EXERCISE FOR YOUR SHOULDER

For the second level you will perform the same exercise as for the first level, but now you will exert more effort. Remember, since this is a test exercise, too much force is not good at all.

Center—IR

Just as before, place the palms of your hands together in front of your body with your elbows bent at a right angle and, with more effort than the first level, push your hands together and Count to 10. Breathe normally.

Interpreting Your Second Level Test Result
Using the Language of Pain

Again, we'll look at all five test results right now and interpret them using the Language of Pain. When you really test a sore part of your body, you will look at only *your* result.

Result 1: You have no pain during the exercise. This is a very good sign. Your body is telling you that it is not experiencing any problem from doing this particular exercise at this increased level of effort. You will be able to progress to the third level of effort for this test exercise.

Result 2: The pain disappears during the exercise. You have pain at first during the test exercise, but the pain disappears during the exercise.

It is likely that the pain was related to lack of flexibility. *PSI* increased your flexibility during the test and the pain went away. You will be able to progress to the third level of effort for this test exercise.

Result 3: The pain is less during the exercise, but it is still there. You have pain during the test exercise; the pain is less intense as you do the exercise, but the pain is still there when you finish the exercise.

It is likely that the pain is related to lack of flexibility and you have not increased your flexibility enough. You may also have some underlying tissue irritation or weakness. To figure this out, you must repeat the same test exercise at the second level of effort for an additional 45 seconds. Then, look once more at your new test result for the second level.

If the pain is less, but some pain remains after you finish the 45-second test exercise, you will be directed back here again. If so, rest 30 seconds and repeat the same 45-second test exercise, in the same position, at the same second level of effort that you just used. Look once more at your new test result for the second level.

If you are directed here a third time, rest for another 30 seconds and do the 45-second test exercise for a third and final time at the second level of effort.

Then, progress to the third level of effort for this test exercise.

Result 4: The pain is unchanged during the exercise. You have pain during the test exercise, and the pain is the same when you finish the exercise.

It is possible that the pain is related to lack of flexibility and you have not increased your flexibility enough. You may also have tissue damage or weakness. To figure this out, you must repeat the same test exercise at the second level of effort for an additional 45 seconds. Then, look once more at your new test result for the second level.

If the pain remains the same during the 45-second test exercise, you will be directed back here. If so, rest 30 seconds and repeat the same 45-second test exercise, in the same position, at the same second level of effort that you just used. Look once more at your new test result for the second level.

If you are directed here a third time, rest for another 30 seconds and do the 45-second test exercise for a third and final time at the second level of effort.

If the pain is the same after three repetitions of the 45-second test exercises at the same level of effort, **STOP!** Something may be wrong. You have completed this test exercise progression. Your test result is 4. If you wish, you can move on to the next first-level test exercise progression.

Result 5: The pain gets worse during the exercise. You have pain as you do the test exercise, and the pain gets worse during the exercise.

STOP! This is a sign of tissue damage or weakness. Your body is telling you to protect these tissues. In the Language of Pain, *increasing pain* means your body is telling you to stop this particular action and to avoid it until damaged tissues heal and are strong enough to perform the action. So stop! Find out what is wrong. You must avoid this action. If you cannot avoid this action during your exercise, don't exercise. If you feel you cannot participate in your sport or dance if you have to avoid this particular action, don't participate! You may get hurt. You should consult an orthopaedic surgeon before you do this particular exercise. You have completed this test exercise progression. Your result is 5. If you wish, you can move on to the next first-level test exercise progression.

THIRD LEVEL 10-SECOND TEST EXERCISE FOR YOUR SHOULDER

For the third level you will perform the same exercise as for the other levels, but now you will exert even more effort—but not maximum effort, because this is still a test exercise. You have the same 5 possible test results for the third level.

Center—IR

Once again, place the palms of your hands together in front of your body with your elbows bent at a right angle and, with more effort than the second level, push your hands together and Count to 10. Breathe normally.

Interpreting Your Third Level Test Result
Using the Language of Pain

Again, we'll look at all 5 test results right now using the Language of Pain. As before, when you really test a sore part of your body, you will look at *your* test result only.

Result 1: You have no pain during the exercise. Congratulations! You passed this exercise test with a Result 1. Your body is telling you that it is not experiencing any problem at all from doing this particular exercise. You should move on to the next first-level test exercise progression, starting again at the first level of effort, and again use the Language of Pain to interpret your result.

The pain or soreness most likely is not related to the action and position of this exercise. It is okay to perform an action like this in the position you tested. The muscles and tendons that perform this action and the joint structures supporting this position are not having a problem.

Result 2: The pain disappears during the exercise. You have pain at first during the test exercise, but the pain disappears during the exercise. Your Result is 2 for this test exercise progression.

Your pain was related to lack of flexibility. *PSI* increased your flexibility during the tests and the pain went away. Move on to the next first-level test exercise progression, starting again at the first level of effort, and again use the Language of Pain to interpret your result.

The pain or soreness related to the action and position of this exercise is possibly due to overuse or poor technique as well as not being warmed up. Since the pain went away after exercise, the muscles and tendons that perform this action and the joint structures supporting this position are not seriously damaged. It is okay to perform an action like this in the position you tested, as long as you adequately warm up first.

If Result 2 is the highest score you get on any of your test exercises, I recommend that you consult a coach or pro about technique in your sport or exercise before any problem develops. Bring a copy of *Natural Flexibility* with you to show the test exercises that bother you.

Result 3: The pain is less during the exercise, but it is still there. You have pain during the test exercise, the pain is less intense as you do the exercise, but the pain is still there when you finish the exercise.

The portion of the pain that disappeared was related to lack of flexibility. The remaining pain may stem from residual lack of flexibility, but you may also have some underlying tissue irritation or weakness. To figure this out, you must repeat the same test exercise at the third level of effort for an additional 45 seconds. Then, look once more at your new test result for the third level.

If the pain is less during the exercise, but some pain remains after you finish the 45-second test exercise, you will be directed back here. If so, rest 30 seconds and repeat the same 45-second test exercise, in the same position, at the same third level of effort that you just used. Look once more at your new test result for the third level.

If you are directed here a third time, rest for another 30 seconds and do the 45-second test exercise for a third and final time at the third level of effort. You will have then completed this test exercise progression. Your Result is 3. Move on to the next first-level test exercise progression, starting again at the first level of effort, and again use the Language of Pain to interpret your result.

After performing three 45-second flexibility exercises, the pain that went away was related to lack of flexibility. The pain that is still there is likely due to some kind of tissue damage. It is best to avoid this action in this position. It is not possible to tell from a single result if the problem lies in the muscles and tendons performing this action, in the joint structures supporting this position, or both. More information is needed to figure this out. As you perform more test exercise progressions, a pattern of pain will emerge. The pattern will tell you if the pain is coming from an action, from a position, or from both.

If Result 3 is the highest you get on any of your test exercises, I recommend that you consult a trainer to check that your fitness and training program are appropriate. You should also consult a coach or pro to ensure you have been using proper technique before the problem gets worse. If the problem does not improve, see your doctor. Bring a copy of *Natural Flexibility* with you to show the test exercises that bother you.

Result 4: The pain is unchanged during the exercise. You have pain during the test exercise, and the pain is the same when you finish the exercise.

You may have tissue damage or weakness. It is possible that the pain is related to lack of flexibility and you have not increased your flexibility enough. To figure this out, you must repeat the same test exercise at the third level for an additional 45 seconds. Then, look once more at your new test result for the third level.

If the pain remains the same during the 45-second test exercise, you will be directed back here. If so, rest 30 seconds and repeat the same 45-second test exercise, in the same position, at the same third level of effort that you just used. Look once more at your new test result for the third level.

If you are directed here a third time, rest for another 30 seconds and do the 45-second test exercise for a third and final time at the third level of effort.

If the pain is the same after three repetitions of the 45-second test exercises at the same level of effort, **STOP!** Something may be wrong. You have completed this test exercise progression. Your Result is 4. Move on to the next first-level test exercise progression, starting again at the first level of effort, and again use the Language of Pain to interpret your result.

The pain or soreness related to the action and position of this exercise is most likely due to tissue damage, because flexibility exercises did not help the pain at all. Repeating this action in this position during your sport or exercise may cause further tissue damage. It is best to avoid this and all other painful actions and positions. It is not possible to tell from a single result if the problem lies in the muscles and tendons performing this action, in the joint structures supporting this position, or both. More information is needed to figure this out. As you perform more test exercise progressions, a pattern of pain will emerge. The pattern will tell you if the pain is coming from an action, from a position, or from both.

If Result 4 is the highest you get on any of your test exercises, I recommend that you consult a certified athletic trainer, licensed physical therapist, or sports medicine doctor before the problem gets worse. Bring a copy of *Natural Flexibility* with you to show the test exercises that bother you.

Result 5: The pain gets worse during the exercise. You have pain as you do the test exercise and the pain gets worse during the exercise.

STOP! This is a sign of tissue damage or weakness. Your body is telling you to protect these tissues. In the Language of Pain, *increasing pain* means your body is telling you to stop this particular action and to avoid it until damaged tissues heal and are strong enough to perform the action. So **STOP!** Find out what is wrong. You have completed this test exercise progression. Your Result is 5. Move on to the next first-level test exercise progression, starting again at the first level of effort, and again use the Language of Pain to interpret your result.

The pain or soreness related to the action and position of this exercise is almost surely based on tissue damage. Performing powerful actions like this in this position, or other positions, during your sport or exercise is likely to cause further tissue damage. Therefore, it is best to stop your sport or exercise. It is not possible to tell from a single result if the problem lies in the muscles and tendons performing this action, in the joint structures supporting this position, or both. More information is needed to figure this out. As you perform more test exercise progressions, a pattern of pain will emerge. The pattern will tell you if the pain is coming from an action, from a position, or both.

If you have any Result 5's on your test exercises, you should consult an orthopaedic surgeon before you resume your sport or exercise. Bring a copy of *Natural Flexibility* with you to show the test exercises that bother you.

Testing Your Shoulder with *PSI*

You have just completed the Center—IR shoulder test exercise progression.

You are now ready for the next test exercise progression in the Center Shoulder Sequence, the Center—ER. The Center—ER test exercise technique employs the same progressive technique as the Center—IR test exercise progression. That is, you perform 3 test exercises at increasing levels of effort. After each test exercise, use the Language of Pain to interpret your results. When you finish the Center—ER test exercise progression, you test with the Center—FL progression, and so on, until you have tested all 6 shoulder actions in the Center Shoulder Sequence position. Use the Language of Pain to interpret each result.

Breathe normally during each of the exercises.

Center Sequence

Move your shoulders so you can place both your hands together comfortably in front of your body. Follow the instructions for each of the following 6 test exercise progressions for the shoulder, using the Language of Pain to interpret each test result.

Center—IR

Place the palms of your hands together with your elbows bent at a right angle and, with a gentle effort, push your hands together and Count to 10. You have already completed the Center—IR test exercise progression, but it is included here for future reference.

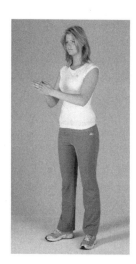

Center—ER

Place your shoulders and arms in the same position that you did for the Center—IR exercise. Clasp your hands together and gently try to pull them apart for 10 seconds. Remember to breathe normally. Use the Language of Pain to interpret your result.

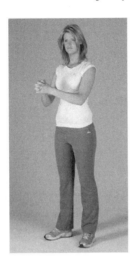

Center—FL

Make a fist with each hand and place the left fist on top of the right. Push your fists together for 10 seconds. Use the Language of Pain to interpret your result. Note: With this sequence, we are actually testing both shoulders at the same time. This test exercise is named for the action

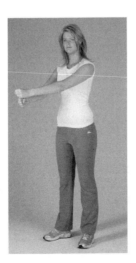

tested with respect to the *right* shoulder. If you wish to refer to the *left* shoulder action for this exercise, it is called EX for **Ex**tension.

Center—EX

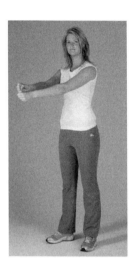

Now switch positions of the hands. Without changing shoulder position, place the right fist on top of the left. Push your fists together for 10 seconds. Use the Language of Pain to interpret your result. Note: This test exercise is named for the action tested with respect to the *right* shoulder. If you wish to refer to the *left* shoulder action for this exercise, it is called FL for **Fl**exion.

Center—AD

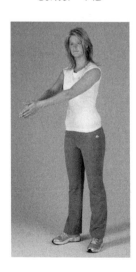

Without changing the position of your shoulders, straighten your elbows out comfortably, but not all the way. Place the palms of your hands together and very gently, push your hands together and Count to 10, like this. Use the Language of Pain to interpret your result.

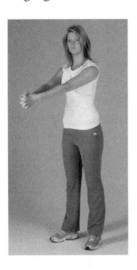

Center—AB

Finally, without changing position at all, clasp your hands again and very gently try to pull your hands apart for 10 seconds. Use the Language of Pain to interpret your result.

To fully test and warm up a sore shoulder you should test the same 6 actions in 4 more shoulder positions. You will see in a moment that this is really quite simple once you get the hang of it. Each sequence will take 3 minutes if there is nothing significantly wrong with your shoulder. Therefore, to fully test your sore shoulder will take about 15 minutes. At the same time, since the testing procedure uses both arms, you will have warmed up both shoulders, elbows, wrists and hands, as well as all the muscles and tendons in both arms and forearms. If you a have problem related to flexibility, it may take a little longer to correct it. So, in a few more minutes, if your completed test results tell you that your shoulder is ready for action, it *will* be ready for action.

Each of the next 4 shoulder positions should be closer to the limit of motion, but don't force the shoulder into an uncomfortable position. There is a Right-Up Sequence, a Left-Up Sequence, a Right-Down Sequence, and a Left-Down Sequence. For each sequence, repeat the same 6 test exercise progressions that you just did in the Center Sequence. *The only difference is the position of your shoulders during the test exercise.*

Your goal is to do each test exercise at three levels of effort without pain. Sometimes you may not be able to reach that goal. From now on, each time you do a new test exercise, you will interpret the test result the same way as the Center—IR, using the Language of Pain.

For reference, here is the Center Sequence on one page:

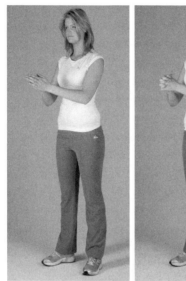
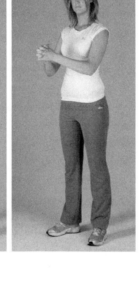

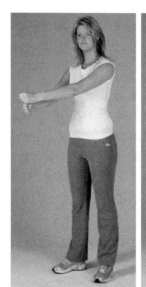
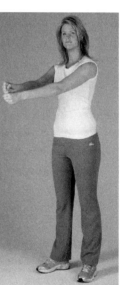

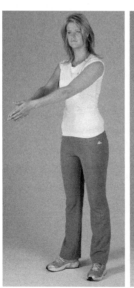
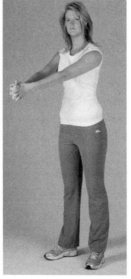

Right-Down Sequence

Move your shoulders so you can place both your hands together as far down and to the right of the front of your body as you comfortably can. Repeat each of the 6 test exercise progressions, using the Language of Pain to interpret each test result. Here is the Right-Down Sequence on one page:

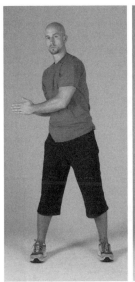
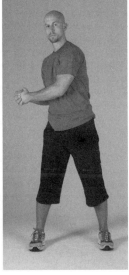

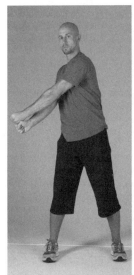
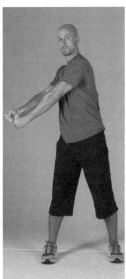

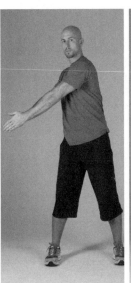
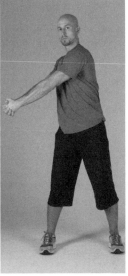

Left-Down Sequence

Move your shoulders so you can place both your hands together as far down and to the left of the front of your body as you comfortably can. Follow the instructions for each of the 6 test exercise progressions for the shoulder, using the Language of Pain to interpret each test result. Here is the Left-Down Sequence on one page:

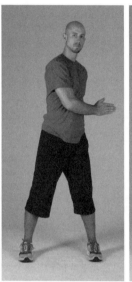
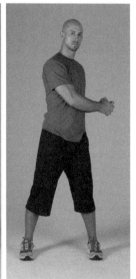
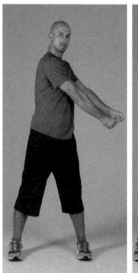
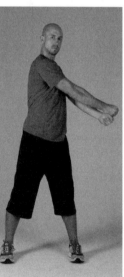
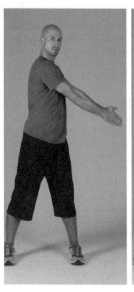
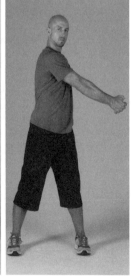

Right-Up Sequence

Move your shoulders so you can place both your hands together as far up and to the right of the front of your body as you comfortably can. Follow the instructions for each of the 6 test exercise progressions for the shoulder, using the Language of Pain to interpret each test result. Here is the Right-Up Sequence on one page:

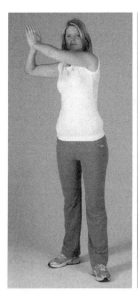
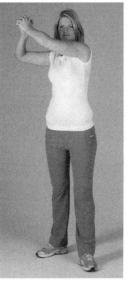
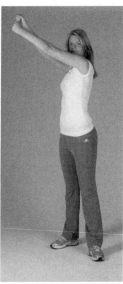
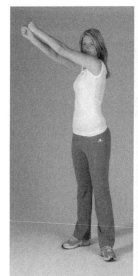
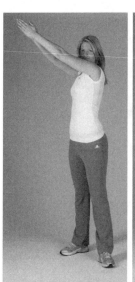
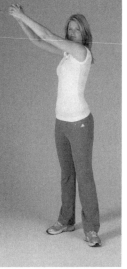

Left-Up Sequence

Move your shoulders so you can place both your hands together as far up and to the left of the front of your body as you comfortably can. Follow the instructions for each of the 6 test exercise progressions for the shoulder, using the Language of Pain to interpret each test result. Here is the Left-Up Sequence on one page:

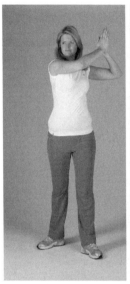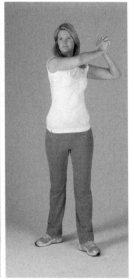

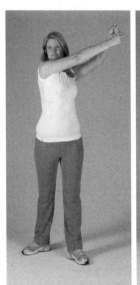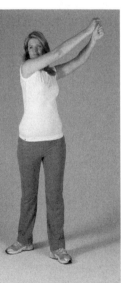

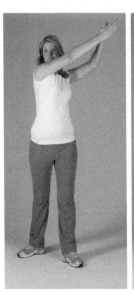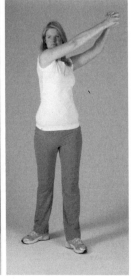

Testing the Rest of Your Body with *PSI*

Remember, testing your right shoulder with *PSI* is just an example of how you can use *PSI*. You can use *PSI* to test and warm up any joint in your body. The logic of *PSI* for your shoulder is the same for any joint. The goal is to test all the muscle actions in the most useful positions of each joint. If your soreness lies in between two joints, you should test both joints. There is no need to test areas of your body that are not sore or tight—regular warm up is enough. We are going to assume you may have a significant problem with your body, so the efforts we demonstrate are in many cases quite gentle compared with athletic or dance activity. At first, try the tests at these lower levels of effort so you become familiar with the actions. **Remember, especially as you study the photos, that you are NOT STRETCHING. Stretching creates exactly the opposite and absolutely incorrect effort.** The muscle you are testing should not be relaxed. The action you are testing is to be resisted so no motion occurs. Do not overpower the action and stretch the muscle. The actions can also be evaluated using a partner, or resistive gym equipment to obtain a test result that is more equivalent to an athletic or dance activity.

The Logic of *PSI* to test any joint:

1. You place your joint in a stable mid-position, away from an extreme limit of its motion.
2. You apply a very gentle effort for 10 seconds without moving. This is a test exercise.
3. You get a result that you interpret with the Language of Pain.
4. You do what your result tells you. Your goal is to perform the test exercise at 3 increasing levels of effort.
5. You do test exercise progressions for each of the main actions, holding the joint in the same position. The set of test exercise progressions done in one joint position make up a joint sequence.
6. Next, you put the joint into a different position, farther from the joint's center of range of motion. You repeat the above test exercises progressions in the new position. Some joints require testing in more positions than others.

You are now going to use the Logic of *PSI* to simultaneously test and warm up all the sore joints of your arms and legs. The shoulder is the most complicated joint, so the test exercises for the other joints will usually be much simpler. These exercises use one side of your body to test the other side. If you prefer, you can use alternative one-sided exercises to test any joint. If you have significant pain, or pain in more than one joint at a time on the same side, such as your wrist and shoulder, you should get some help from a licensed physical therapist or doctor before you start. Bring a copy of *Natural Flexibility* with you to discuss the test exercises. Any certified athletic trainer or physical therapist should be able to help you to substitute exercises if necessary.

Soreness and pain in your neck and back are covered in Chapter 7: Your Chiropractor in Your Pocket.

NATURAL FLEXIBILITY TECHNIQUE:
Testing Your Elbow

Your elbow performs 2 actions: **FL**exion and **EX**tension. Both actions will be tested in 3 sequence positions, the Center position, the fully flexed position, and finally in the fully extended position. As you did with the shoulder, you will perform each test exercise at 3 levels of effort, using the Language of Pain to interpret each test result. We will demonstrate the exercises for the right elbow.

Center Elbow Sequence

Bend your elbow to a right angle. Follow the instructions for the **FL** and **EX** test exercise progressions, using the Language of Pain to interpret each test result.

Center—FL

As you try to bend your right elbow further, resist with your left hand, so no motion occurs. Use the Language of Pain to interpret each test result.

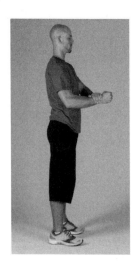

As you try to straighten your right elbow further, resist with your left hand, so no motion occurs. Use the Language of Pain to interpret each test result.

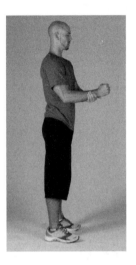

Flexed Elbow Sequence

Bend your elbow as far as it will comfortably go. Follow the instructions for the **FL** and **EX** test exercise progressions, using the Language of Pain to interpret each test result.

Flexed—FL

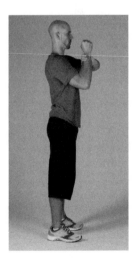

Flexed—EX

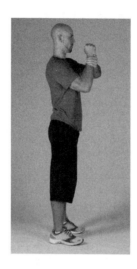

Extended Elbow Sequence

Straighten your elbow as far as it will comfortably go. Follow the instructions for the **FL** and **EX** test exercise progressions, using the Language of Pain to interpret each test result.

Extended—FL

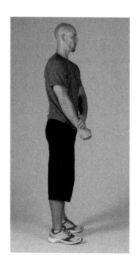

Extended—EX

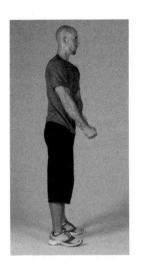

NATURAL FLEXIBILITY TECHNIQUE:
Testing Your Forearm

Technically, your forearm is not a joint, but it does have two joints at either end with 2 actions: Pronation and Supination. Both actions will be tested in 3 positions, the Center position, the fully pronated position, and the fully supinated position. Interpret your results using the Language of Pain. We will demonstrate the exercises for the right forearm.

Center Forearm Sequence

Bend your elbow to a right angle and turn your wrist so your thumb points up. Follow the instructions for the **P** and **S** test exercise progressions, using the Language of Pain to interpret each test result.

Center—P

As you try to turn your right forearm so palm turns down, resist with your left hand, so no motion occurs. Use the Language of Pain to interpret each test result.

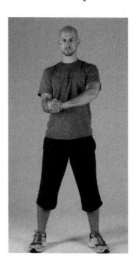

Center—S

As you try to turn your right forearm so palm turns up, resist with your left hand, so no motion occurs. Use the Language of Pain to interpret each test result.

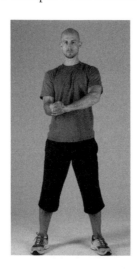

Pronated Forearm Sequence

Bend your elbow to a right angle and turn your wrist so your palm faces almost all the way down. Follow the instructions for the **P** and **S** test exercise progressions, using the Language of Pain to interpret each test result.

Pronated—P

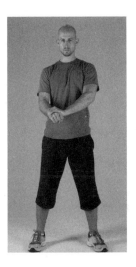

Pronated—S

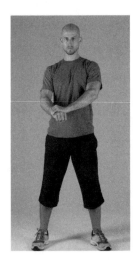

Supinated Forearm Sequence

Bend your elbow to a right angle and turn your wrist so your palm faces almost all the way up. Follow the instructions for the **P** and **S** test exercise progressions, using the Language of Pain to interpret each test result.

Supinated—P

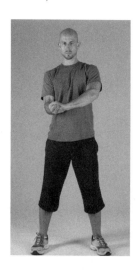

Supinated—S

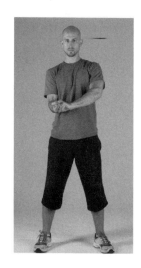

Testing Your Wrist

We will test 4 wrist actions: **Flexion**, **Extension**, **Radial Deviation**, and **Ulnar Deviation**. **Flexion** and **Extension** actions will be tested in Center position, the fully extended position, and finally in the fully flexed position. **Radial Deviation** and **Ulnar Deviation** actions will be tested in the Neutral position, then fully deviated to either side. As you did with the shoulder, you will perform each test exercise at 3 levels of effort, using the Language of Pain to interpret each test result. We will demonstrate the exercises for the right wrist.

Center Wrist Sequence

Bend your elbow to a right angle with your wrist turned so your thumb side is up. Follow the instructions for the **FL** and **EX** test exercise progressions, using the Language of Pain to interpret each test result.

Center—FL

Make a fist with your right hand. As you try to bend your right wrist, resist with your left hand, so no motion occurs. Use the Language of Pain to interpret each test result.

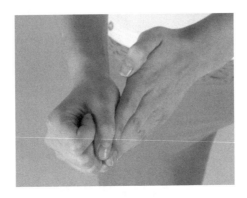

Center—EX

As you try to straighten your right wrist, resist with your left hand, so no motion occurs. Use the Language of Pain to interpret each test result.

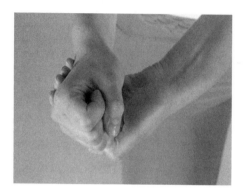

Flexed Wrist Sequence

Bend your wrist as far as it will comfortably go. Follow the instructions for the **FL** and **EX** test exercise progressions, as you just did for the Center position. Use the Language of Pain to interpret each test result.

Flexed—FL

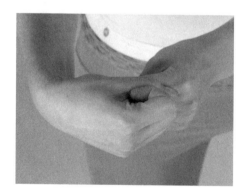

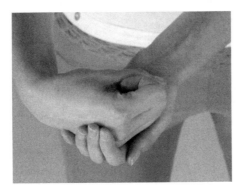

Extended Wrist Sequence

Bend your wrist back as far as it will comfortably go. Follow the instructions for the **FL** and **EX** test exercise progressions, as you just did for the Center position. Use the Language of Pain to interpret each test result.

Extended—FL

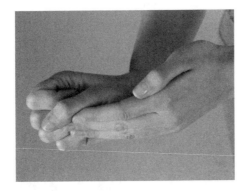

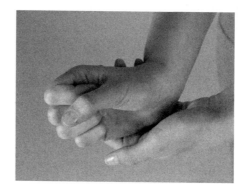

Neutral Wrist Sequence

Bend your elbow to a right angle and turn your wrist so your palm faces down. Follow the instructions for the **RD** and **UD** test exercise progressions, using the Language of Pain to interpret each test result.

Neutral—RD

As you try to angle your right hand to the thumb side, resist with your left hand, so no motion occurs. Use the Language of Pain to interpret each test result.

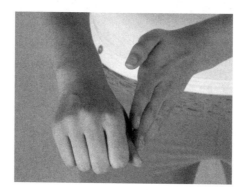

Neutral—UD

As you try to angle your right hand toward the little finger side, resist with your left hand, so no motion occurs. Use the Language of Pain to interpret each test result.

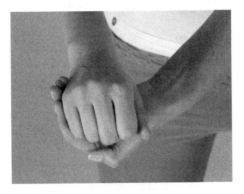

Radially Deviated Wrist Sequence

With your palm facing down, angle your wrist and hand toward the thumb side as far as comfortable. Follow the instructions for the **RD** and **UD** test exercise progressions, using the Language of Pain to interpret each test result.

Radially Deviated—RD

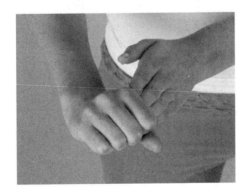

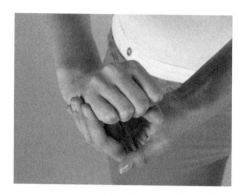

Ulnarly Deviated Wrist Sequence

With your palm facing down, angle your wrist and hand toward the little finger side as far as comfortable. Follow the instructions for the **RD** and **UD** test exercise progressions, using the Language of Pain to interpret each test result.

Ulnarly Deviated—RD

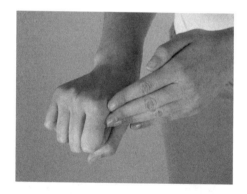

Ulnarly Deviated—UD

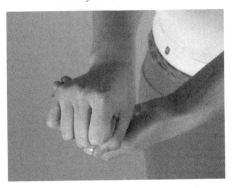

NATURAL FLEXIBILITY TECHNIQUE:
Testing Your Fingers And Thumbs

Each finger performs 4 basic actions: **FL**exion, **EX**tension, **AD**duction and **AB**duction. As you did with the shoulder, you will perform each test exercise at 3 levels of effort, using the Language of Pain to interpret each test result. We are testing the right index finger. All the fingers and thumbs can be tested the same way.

Center Finger Sequence

Let your finger rest comfortably. Follow the instructions for the **FL** and **EX** test exercise progressions, using the Language of Pain to interpret each test result.

Center—FL

As you try to bend your finger further, resist with your left hand, so no motion occurs. Use the Language of Pain to interpret each test result.

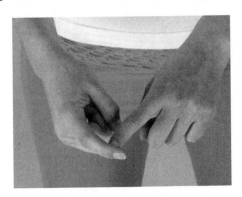

Center—EX

As you try to straighten your right finger further, resist with your left hand, so no motion occurs. Use the Language of Pain to interpret each test result.

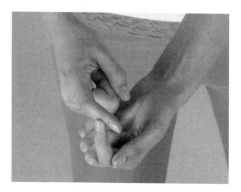

Flexed Finger Sequence

Bend your finger as far as it will comfortably go. Follow the instructions for the **FL** and **EX** test exercise progressions, using the Language of Pain to interpret each test result.

Flexed—FL

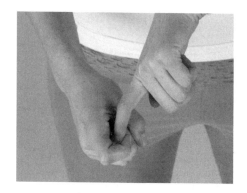

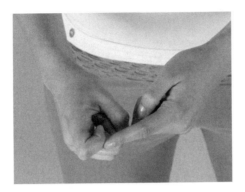

Extended Finger Sequence

Straighten your finger as far as it will comfortably go. Follow the instructions for the **FL** and **EX** test exercise progressions, using the Language of Pain to interpret each test result.

Extended—FL

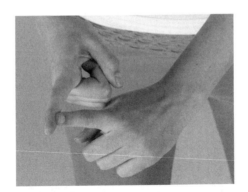

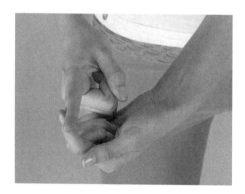

Neutral Right Thumb Sequence

Let your right thumb rest comfortably as shown. Follow the instructions for the **AB** and **AD** test exercise progressions, using the Language of Pain to interpret each test result. Like every other joint, the thumb can be tested in more extreme positions than this to evaluate pain. The fingers can be tested the same way.

Neutral—AB

As you try to move your thumb away from your palm, resist with your left hand, so no motion occurs. Use the Language of Pain to interpret each test result.

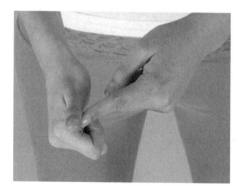

Neutral—AD

As you try to move your thumb closer to your palm, resist with your left hand, so no motion occurs. Use the Language of Pain to interpret each test result.

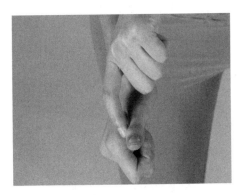

NATURAL FLEXIBILITY TECHNIQUE:
Testing Your Hips

The hip has 6 actions like the shoulder, and 5 positions, but the range of motion of the hip is not as great. Each test exercise progression is a set of three 10-second exercises. Use the Language of Pain to interpret your results. Remember to breathe normally. We are going to test the right hip. We have demonstrated the exercises using the arms or floor for resistance. Alternatively, you could use a partner or resistive gym equipment. It is always important to accurately reproduce the resisted hip action you are testing.

Center Sequence

Sit in a chair so you can place both your feet together comfortably in front of your body. Your right hip should be bent as you sit. Follow the instructions for each of the following 6 test exercise progressions for the shoulder, using the Language of Pain to interpret each test result.

Center—IR

Try to slide your right foot further to the right, but resist the action using your left foot. You should feel a rotation at the right hip called Internal Rotation.

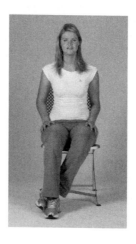

Center—ER

Try to slide your right foot to the left, but again resist the action using your left foot. You should feel a rotation at the right hip called External Rotation.

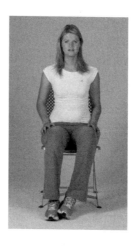

Center—FL

Try to lift your right thigh, so the hip tries to bend forward, but resist the action using your hand. The right hip action you are testing is **FL**exion.

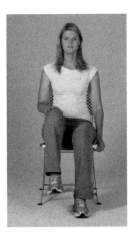

Center—EX

Push against the floor with your right foot, as though you were going to get up from the chair, but do not move. The action should try to straighten the hip and is called **EX**tension.

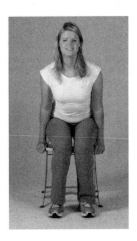

Center—AD

Try to move your right knee toward the left knee so the hip swings to your left, but resist the action using your hand. The right hip action you are testing is **AD**duction.

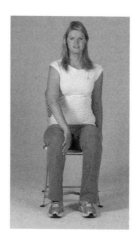

Center—AB

Finally, try to move your right knee away from the left knee so the hip swings to your right, but resist the action using your hand. The right hip action you are testing is **AB**duction.

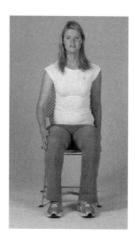

Each of the next 4 hip positions should be closer to the limit of motion, but don't force the hip into an uncomfortable position. There is a Flexed Sequence, an Extended Sequence, an Adducted Sequence, and an Abducted Sequence. For each sequence, repeat the same six 10-second test exercise progressions that you just did in the Center Sequence. *The only difference is the position of your hips during the test exercise.*

Your goal is to do each test exercise at three levels of effort without pain. Sometimes you may not be able to reach that goal. Each time you do a new test exercise, you will interpret the test result the same way, using the Language of Pain.

For reference, here is the Center Sequence on one page:

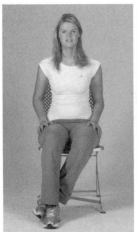
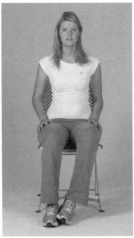
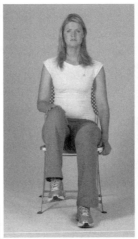
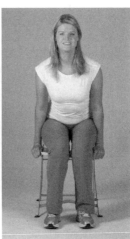
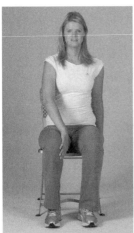
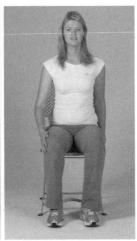

Flexed Sequence

Lift your right leg at the hip, as far as you comfortably can, keeping your right knee bent. Repeat each of the 6 test exercise progressions, using the Language of Pain to interpret each test result. Here is the Flexed Sequence on one page:

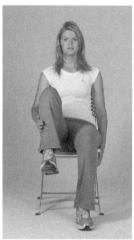
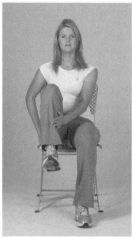

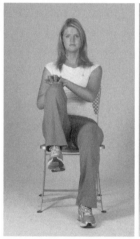
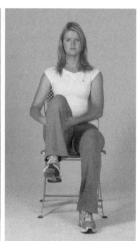

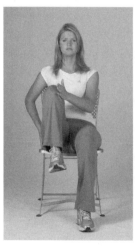
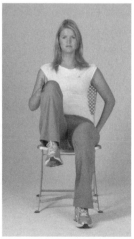

Extended Sequence

Stand up and straighten your right leg at the hip, as far as you comfortably can, keeping your right knee straight. Repeat each of the 6 test exercise progressions, using the Language of Pain to interpret each test result. Here is the Extended Sequence on one page:

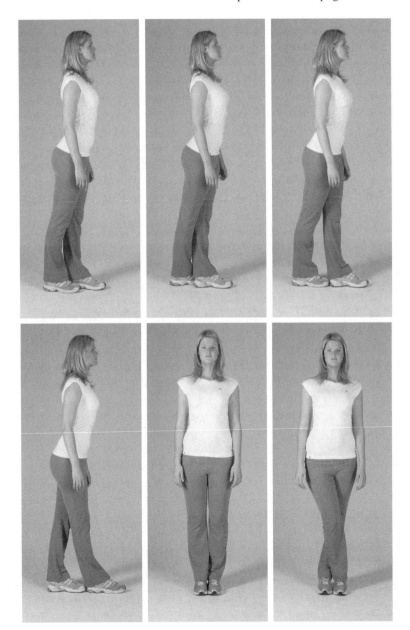

Adducted Sequence

While you sit on the floor, bend your right hip and knee comfortably. Move your right knee as close to your left knee as you comfortably can. Repeat each of the 6 test exercise progressions, using the Language of Pain to interpret each test result. Here is the Adducted Sequence on one page:

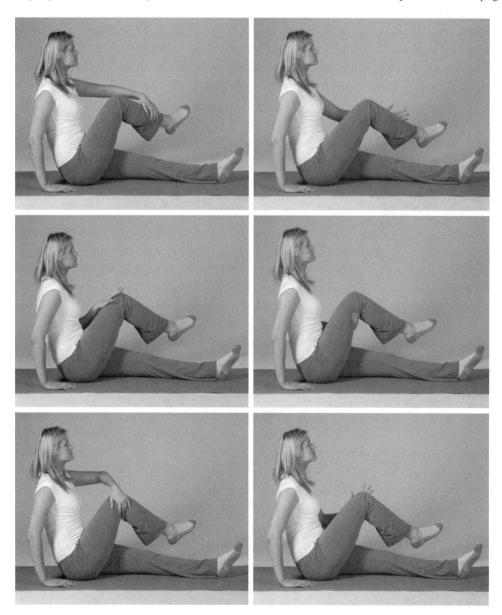

Abducted Sequence

While you sit on the floor, bend your right hip and knee comfortably. Move your right knee as far away from your left knee as you comfortably can. Repeat each of the 6 test exercise progressions, using the Language of Pain to interpret each test result. Here is the Abducted Sequence on one page:

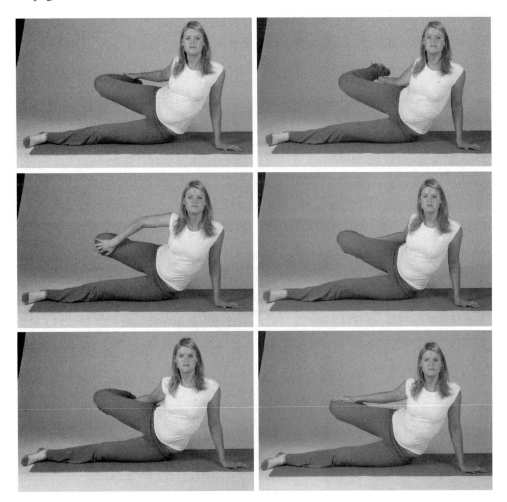

NATURAL FLEXIBILITY TECHNIQUE:

Testing Your Knees

Traditionally, the knee is said to have 2 actions, **FL**exion and **EX**tension. We will also test 2 more actions, Internal Rotation and External Rotation. We will test the right knee in 3 sequence positions.

Center Sequence

Sit in a chair so you can place both your feet together comfortably in front of your body. Your right hip and knee should be bent as you sit. Follow the instructions for each of the following 4 test exercise progressions for the knee, using the Language of Pain to interpret each test result.

Center—IR

Keeping your right foot on the floor, try to rotate your right foot and leg counter-clockwise, but resist the action using your left foot against the inside of your right forefoot. You should feel a resisted rotation at the right knee called Internal Rotation.

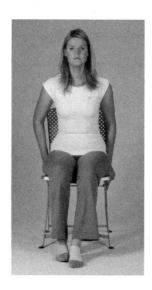

Center—ER

Keeping your right foot on the floor, try to rotate your right foot and leg clockwise, but resist the action using your left foot against the outside of your right forefoot. You should feel a resisted rotation at the right knee called **External Rotation**.

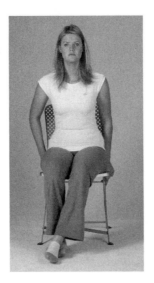

Center—FL

Keeping your right foot on the floor, try to bend your right knee backward, but resist the action using your left foot against the back of the heel of your right foot. The resisted right knee action you are testing is **FL**exion.

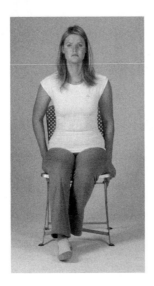

Keeping your right foot on the floor, try to straighten your right knee, but resist the action using your left foot against the front of your right foot. The resisted right knee action you are testing is called **EX**tension.

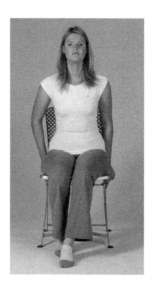

For reference, here is the Center Sequence on one page:

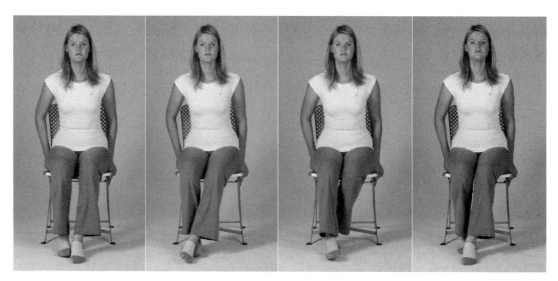

Extended Sequence

Stand up and straighten your right leg at the hip and knee. Keeping your right knee straight, repeat each of the 4 test exercise progressions, using the Language of Pain to interpret each test result. Here is the Extended Sequence on one page:

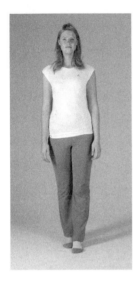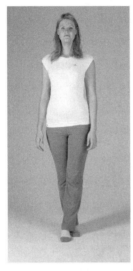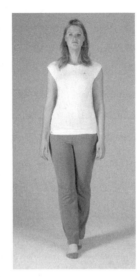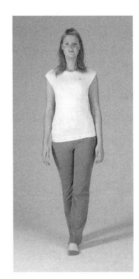

Flexed Sequence

Lift your right leg at the hip and bend your right knee as far as you comfortably can. Repeat each of the 4 test exercise progressions, using the Language of Pain to interpret each test result. Here is the Flexed Sequence on one page:

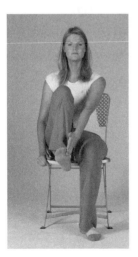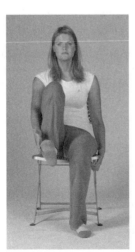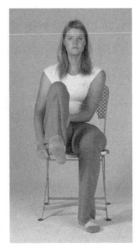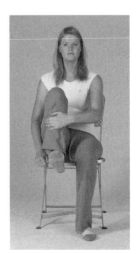

NATURAL FLEXIBILITY TECHNIQUE:

Testing Your Ankles, Feet, and Toes

The ankle and foot have many joints, and hence many actions and positions. We will test a few combined actions. We are assuming you may have a significant problem with your foot or ankle, so these efforts are quite gentle compared with regular standing or walking. The actions can also be evaluated using a partner, or resistive gym equipment to obtain a test result that is more equivalent to an athletic or dance activity.

Dorsiflexion

Sit on a chair with your ankle in a comfortable position on the floor. Try to bend your right ankle up, but resist the action using your hand or left foot against the top of your right foot. You should feel a resisted action at the right ankle called **Dorsiflexion**.

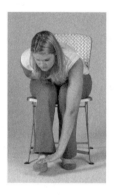

Plantarflexion

Sit on a chair with your ankle in a comfortable position on the floor. Try to bend your right ankle down, but resist the action using your hand or left foot against the bottom of your right foot. You should feel a resisted action at the right ankle called **Plantarflexion**.

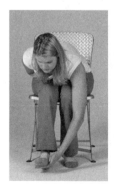

Inversion

Grip your right forefoot with your left hand. Try to bend the sole of your right foot inward, but resist the action using your left hand against the left side of your foot. The resisted action you are testing is **Inversion**.

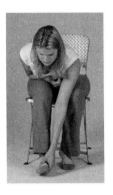

Eversion

Grip your right forefoot with your right hand. Try to bend the sole of your right foot outward, but resist the action using your right hand against the right side of your foot. The resisted action you are testing is **Eversion**.

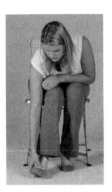

The toes work a lot like the fingers, but obviously with less emphasis on dexterity and more on weight-bearing. We demonstrate the right great toe, but all toes have the same actions.

Dorsiflexion

Sit on a chair with your right foot in a comfortable position on the floor. Try to bend your toe up, but resist the action using your hand against the top of your toe. You should feel a resisted action at the toe called **Dorsiflexion**.

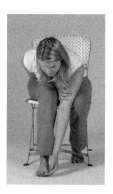

Plantarflexion

Sit on a chair with your right foot in a comfortable position on the floor. Try to bend your toe down, but resist the action using your hand against the bottom of your toe. You should feel a resisted action at the toe called **Plantarflexion**.

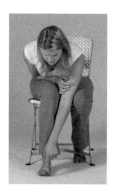

YOUR RESULTS

You should already realize that higher result scores are not as good as lower result scores. The higher the score, the more likely tissue damage is causing your soreness. These higher scores should pinpoint the actions and positions causing the soreness. If your soreness is related to your sport or exercise activity, you will already have a good basis to figure out exactly what activities are responsible and what to do about it. This is only intended to be a guide, not a personal treatment plan. You may be wrong in thinking your sport or exercise is what is causing your pain. If you have severe pain or pain that continues for more than a few days, pain that gets worse, pain that bothers you at night, or pain that has other symptoms associated with it such as fever, weakness, numbness, swelling, deformity, discoloration, or anything else that bothers or concerns you, SEE YOUR DOCTOR!

Higher result scores primarily during the same action, but in different positions, are most likely caused by a problem with a muscle or tendon, because muscles and tendons perform approximately the same actions in the different positions we tested. If instead you have higher result scores primarily in a particular position, you most likely have something wrong with the joint surface, or an impingement (something catching, like a cartilage or small tendon tear). Again, this is a useful simplification. Some structures, like chondromalacia of the joint surface, come under stress in only certain positions, and will show up as problems in one certain positions only. Others, like the bone, come under stress in all positions. Fractures are likely to produce problems in many positions and with many actions.

With this in mind, you can once again look at all your final test sequence results and understand better what they mean. The same patterns of high result scores affecting actions, positions, or both, can occur when you test all parts of your body and the principles are the same.

Remember, I am not trying to diagnose your problem. I am simply trying to give you an idea about what might be going wrong so you can take appropriate action to protect and help yourself. You need a real orthopaedic surgeon doing a real orthopaedic examination to get a real orthopaedic diagnosis. I am a real orthopaedic surgeon, but I am not examining you and I am not diagnosing you with these test exercises!

A Few Tips

You may have been able to do a test exercise at a lower level of effort without pain but then have pain at a higher level. This means the tissues are not strong enough to handle the higher level of effort. You may still perform actions like this exercise during your sport or dance *provided the pain does not get worse and you are certain to apply less effort than you did during the test that provoked symptoms,* but you should first get clearance from a certified athletic trainer or licensed physical therapist. Bring a copy of *Natural Flexibility* with you to discuss the exercises you'd like to do.

If the result of your test exercise directed you to STOP, then you cannot progress to the next level of testing with this particular exercise. You are free to try any other test exercise. If more than one type of test exercise progression gives you a STOP result, it is unlikely you will be able to perform actions like these during your sport or dance without significant risk. Consult an orthopaedic surgeon. Bring a copy of *Natural Flexibility* with you and show the doctor the test exercises that bother you.

Testing using both your arms or legs at the same time is convenient and saves time—you are warming up both as you do the tests. This technique may alert you to problems in some other area than the one being tested. In such cases, you may wish to test the new area with exercises specific for that joint. Some of you may already have pain or a known problem that prevents you from doing the exercises this way. Testing your body with isometric exercise does not require use of both arms or legs. If you have problems doing the test exercises using both arms or legs, consult a licensed physical therapist for assistance with the exercises. Bring a copy of *Natural Flexibility* with you and show the therapist the test exercises that you wish to do.

The Proof of the Pudding

If you started out with pain and you no longer have pain, you now know that you are ready for your exercise, sport, or dance. If you still have pain, you know what you can do and what you can't do with your body. You already have a good idea about the nature of the problem and why you have it. Finally, you know whom you should consult for help.

How does that compare with stretching?

Chapter 7

Your Chiropractor *in your* Pocket

NECK AND BACK pain are among the most disabling conditions in our nation. Despite intensive research and an incredible investment of human resources, the problem continues to plague millions of Americans. Neck and back pain have not been cured by anything someone can do to you. No medication, no manipulation, no surgical procedure treats most neck and back pain better than you can all by yourself with a few minutes of exercise.

AN OUNCE OF PREVENTION . . .

Common neck and back pain is usually due to sprains of varying degrees of severity and resultant muscle spasm. Other causes of neck and back pain are much less common, but may be serious. If you already have neck or back pain, you should confirm your diagnosis with your doctor before you begin, because certain conditions, such as a spinal fracture or ruptured disks, require special precautions. If you have common neck or back pain, and you do the following exercises every day before you get out of bed, you will do as much as anyone can to prevent future neck and back injury, and to relieve pain you already have. Furthermore, if symptoms return during the day, you can simply lie down on the floor and do the exercises all over again, with immediate benefit that will be just as helpful as any surgery, therapy, or adjustments. You can just pull them out of your pocket, so to speak, without an appointment, without your insurance card, without pre-approval. These exercises must be done every morning before you start your day.

You are about to learn exercises that will get rid of the stiffness of your spine by gently squeezing the excess fluid out of your disks. These exercises will also encourage the structural molecules in your spinal supporting tissues to rearrange themselves, making you more flexible. They will also relieve muscle spasm. All this takes at least a few minutes to happen. If you rush, if you exert too much force while you do the exercises, you could make matters worse. It is very important to understand the gentle nature of these exercises. The key is to listen to your body. To better understand your body's Language of Pain, you may wish to refer to Chapter 6, "When You're Sore." When you have pain as you begin an exercise, the pain should lessen as you count to 10 slowly, or the exercise is not right for you. Sometimes you need to decrease the amount of force you are using until you sense improvement. Sometimes the exercise is simply not right for your condition. Your back or neck pain may not be due to a straightforward disk displacement. If you have pain radiating down your arm or leg, numbness, or weakness, you may have a ruptured disk with nerve impingement. You need to consult your doctor about this kind of problem.

Do not expect to be cured by these exercises. They are designed to make you feel better and help you to increase your activity level for the day more safely. They have tremendous preventative value if you do them regularly before you get hurt, or at least before you get hurt the next time. Recovery from intervertebral disk displacements can take weeks to months, so be patient. The exercises I am about to teach you will replace a group of harmful stretches, including two that are particularly misunderstood as being fitness indicators: the "sit and reach" stretch and the "toe touch" stretch.

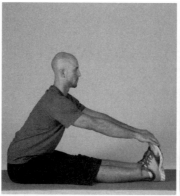 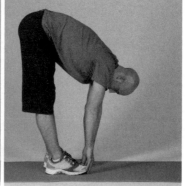

Instead, here are a few safe and effective exercises for your neck and back.

HELPING YOUR NECK AND BACK
Isometric Flexion Exercise: Level 1

SET UP: The first exercise should be done every morning: lie on your back, hips and knees bent, feet on the bed. Move your pillow to the side, out of the way. Put your hands under your pelvis, like this, to straighten your lower back and load the intervertebral disks more evenly.

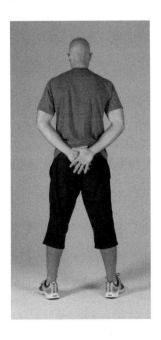

NATURAL FLEXIBILITY TECHNIQUE

1. Slowly, bend your hips and lift your knees up toward your chest, not all the way, just to a comfortable position. At the same time, lift your head not more than one inch from the bed, looking straight at the ceiling all the time. *This is a very gentle exercise.* Do not force it.

2. Count to 10 slowly, one second per count. If you have increasing pain, bend your knees more to decrease the stress. If you still have increasing pain, you should stop here and confirm with your doctor or therapist that it is okay to continue. Most of the time, if your pain is getting worse, it is because you are not being gentle enough: be gentler and try again. If you have pain at the beginning, but it does not get worse,

that is okay. Remember to breathe naturally during the exercise. Your heart will pump blood to your muscles and we want that blood to have plenty of oxygen in it. So breathe!

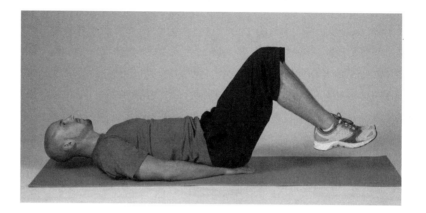

3. After 10 seconds, put your head and feet down again. Rest for 10 seconds. Then, repeat the exercise. If you feel up to it, increase the count to 20 seconds. Keep looking at the ceiling with your head lifted no more than about one inch from the bed (to make sure you do not bend your neck) and keep your knees bent toward your chest gently. Rest for 10 seconds. Throughout the exercise, you should be breathing naturally—do not hold your breath. Again, if you have increasing pain, stop. If you still have some of the pain you started with, don't be dismayed. You probably will feel a tension and sense of fatigue in your neck, as well as a tightness or pressure as you do the exercise. This should lessen considerably and eventually disappear as you rest. If your neck becomes too tired, put your head back on the bed for part of the exercise, as you need to. Eventually your neck will become stronger. Remember to breathe naturally.

4. Repeat the exercise for thirty seconds. Rest. After this, you may hold the exercise for as long as you wish, up to a minute. Breathe naturally. Your back tension may decrease as you do the exercise, until you reach a plateau. Your neck may become too tired to continue. Either way, that is your limit. It is important to remember not to force your body. Do not make a strenuous effort. This is not a "No pain, no gain" exercise.

Meanwhile, what have you been accomplishing with these exercises? At night, as you sleep and your body relaxes, fluids begin to accumulate in the tissues that support you during the day. Large supporting molecules change their shape and position and become knotted together. This makes the tissues in your spine swell and become stiffer. Any pressure on these tissues will be transmitted to sore areas and cause pain, as well as increased risk for injury if excess force is applied to the area. The exercises you are doing, over several minutes, will gently squeeze that fluid out of the tissues and rearrange the structural molecules, so that your tissues become more flexible. When you finally get up, the pressure placed on your spine should not hurt as much. Placing your hands behind your pelvis tilts the lumbar spine forward, loading the disk more evenly. If you already have a damaged disk, this may help to gently centralize the disk.

During sleep, the blood flow to your muscles decreases. If you have a disk or pinched nerve problem in your back or neck, these cold muscles are prone to tightness and spasm. With these exercises, your muscles will warm up as muscle blood flow increases and the spasm will disappear.

As you continue to do these exercises over several weeks, your body will also become stronger. The next exercises use slightly more force (now that your body is warmed up slightly) to do the same things. Ready?

Isometric Flexion Exercise: Level 2

SET UP: The next exercise starts out like the first. Place your hands under your pelvis.

NATURAL FLEXIBILITY TECHNIQUE

1. Instead of lifting your legs with your hips and knees bent as much as before, keep your hips and knees a little straighter. Your upper body should come a little further from the bed. As it does, keep looking at the ceiling. Your neck will bend back (extend) a little more as you do this.

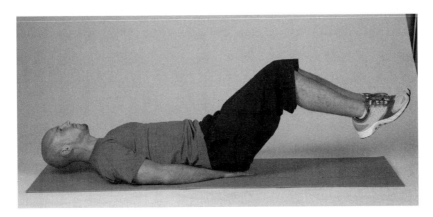

If you have increasing pain in your neck, you are bending it back or forward to much. If you have increasing pain in your back or down your legs, you have straightened your knees too much. Count to 10, then rest for 10 seconds.

2. Repeat for twenty seconds and rest for twenty.

3. Then repeat for thirty seconds and rest. If you are up for it, do one more final repetition for as long as you wish up to 1 minute. During this final rep, you may straighten your knees out slowly as much as you feel good about doing. You may bend them again as much as you want if you tire. Just like before, if your neck becomes too tired, you may rest it on the bed for a portion of the exercises as much as you need to until your neck muscles become stronger. Breathe—don't hold your breath during the exercise.

Dynamic Flexion Exercise

SET UP: Start the same way, lying on your back in bed, hands under your pelvis. Bend your hips and knees a little. You may hold them as straight as you feel comfortable, based on the previous exercise. Lift your head a little, looking at the ceiling. Do not bend your neck.

NATURAL FLEXIBILITY TECHNIQUE

1. Lift both legs up as high as you feel comfortable. There is no reason to force them to go as high as possible.

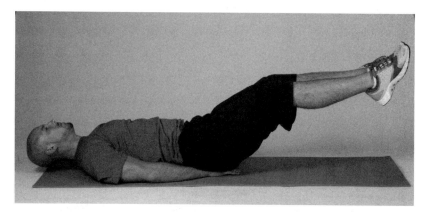

2. As you lift your legs, slightly turn your head to the right. Again, there is no reason to go as far as you can, just as far as you are comfortable.

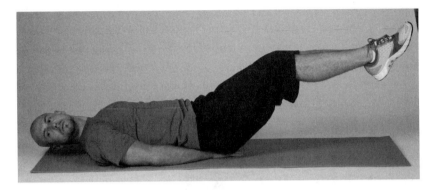

3. Put your legs almost all the way down again, but don't touch the bed, and turn your head straight ahead again, without putting it down. Immediately repeat the exercise with your head turned to the left. Keep your head one inch from the bed at all times. Do not force your neck at all. If you have increasing pain in your neck, you have turned it too much.

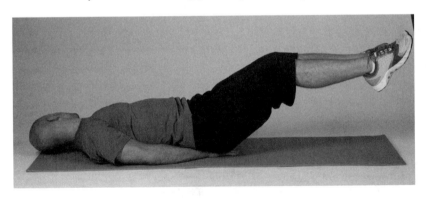

4. Again put your legs almost all the way down without touching the bed and turn your head straight ahead again, without putting it down.
5. Do as many reps as you feel comfortable doing.
6. Stop and relax whenever you need to.

Your goal, after about six weeks of trying, is at least 30 reps, but you may go for as many as you wish. Your abdominal muscles will strengthen and firm with time, and your posture will improve.

Isometric Trunk Rotation Exercise

SET UP: This is the last exercise of the set. Start in the same basic position lying on your back in bed, hands under your pelvis. Bend your hips and knees as much as comfortable (more than the last exercise). Lift your head a little, looking at the ceiling. Cross your legs at the ankles, so that one is over the other.

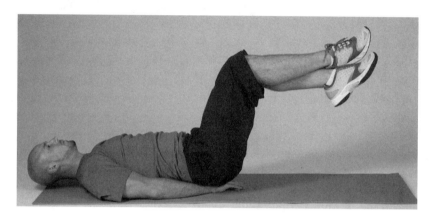

1. Rotate your hips so your knees lean to the right a little, keeping your knees bent. Lean as far as you feel comfortable. Count to 10.

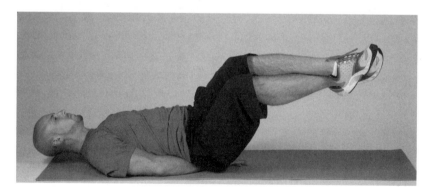

2. Now lean to the left, still with your knees bent comfortably. Count to 10.

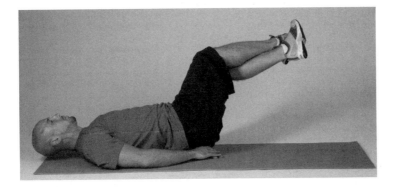

3. Now lean again to the right, but this time, straighten your knees a little bit. You will feel yourself lean further automatically. Hold this new position for a count of ten.

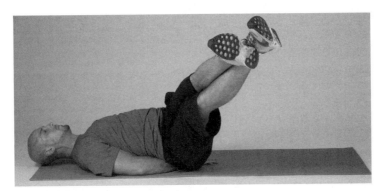

4. Then lean to the left with your knees bent the same amount, for a count of ten.

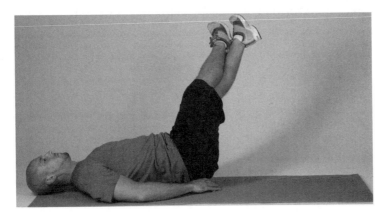

You will feel the rotator muscles in your lower back and abdomen working to hold your legs up. As you straighten your knees, they have to work a little harder. If you find yourself tiring, bend your knees a little more. Do not lose control. Keep your knees bent as much as you need for control. Do not let your legs fall onto the bed as you lean to the side. Do not relax your muscles as you lean to the side. This is not a stretch!

5. Now face forward, put your head and legs down, and relax.

USEFUL TRICKS

Getting into bed can be tough with low back pain. The kind of bed and height of the bed are a factor here. High, stiff beds are much easier to deal with. Low water beds are the worst. I recommend placing a ¾ inch-thick piece of plywood between your mattress and box spring to support the mattress.

Once you are in bed, all is not won. You will still have trouble turning from one side to the other during the night. This is best accomplished with your knees bent. If you are lying on your back, you will probably find one or both of the following two tricks a life saver. Place a small folded towel or pillow case under your pelvis, NOT under your spine, in exactly the same place you placed your hands during your exercises, to straighten your lower lumbar spine. The thickness and placement of the towel is crucial. If you have common low back pain, you should have **immediate and almost complete relief** if you place the towel in the right spot. If not, experiment with placing the towel in a slightly different location. Very often, the towel has been folded too thick or it is too big a towel. It could be too thin. About ¾ inch is satisfactory. Place a pillow under your knees to keep them bent. Sometimes, you only need the pillow under one knee. When you want to lie on your side, take the folded towel from behind your pelvis. Place it under your waist. Place the pillow between your knees, but keep them bent.

If your neck is the problem, the same kind of folded towel is sometimes much better than your pillow. High pillows are usually a nuisance.

Some people are so miserable with their back pain that they cannot get into bed, or cannot get comfortable once they are in bed. Sometimes it is worthwhile to lie on the floor, next to a bed or couch, your knees bent, and with your legs on the couch, using the same technique with the folded towel to straighten your lower lumbar spine.

WASHING UP, BRUSHING YOUR TEETH, SHAVING, AND. . . .

Avoid bending over at your waist if you have low back pain. If you have pain down your leg from your back, a small footstool under your affected leg can make these obligations doable. This is true also of many other activities that require standing in one position, such as washing dishes. Even sitting can be helped with a small lift under one foot, usually the side that is worse. Be careful to sit back all the way. Don't slouch. Sitting at the dinner table can be managed this way too. In addition, keep one forearm against the edge of the table for support. After dinner, if your neck is a problem, a cervical collar worn until you go to bed can relax muscles that have been in spasm all day. Neck pain becomes a real pain in the neck during socialization. Avoid nodding your head or turning it from side to side during conversations.

LIFTING, DRIVING, AND THE REST OF YOUR LIFE

Your physical therapist can be most helpful in teaching proper body mechanics and adjusting activity levels to your individual needs. In general, avoid bending, twisting or turning with your neck or back. If you drop something, this is a good way to pick it up.

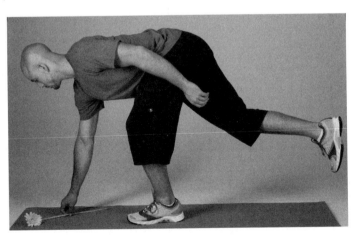

Common neck and back pain often take many weeks to disappear, only to reappear every few years. Although you should gain immediate relief from the exercises you have just learned, their most important benefit is to prevent this pattern of recurrence in the future. This benefit will accrue only if you do these exercises every morning before you start your day. These are preparatory exercises. The effect lasts only a few hours. Although you will strengthen your spine as you continue to do them, it is not the increase in strength that is most helpful in prevention. It is the morning preparation of the spine for what lies ahead during the day.

Appendix

Suggested Readings and References

Ahmad, C.S., A.M. Clark, N. Heilmann, et al. 2006. Effect of gender and maturity on quadriceps-to-hamstring strength ratio and anterior cruciate ligament laxity. *American Journal of Sports Medicine* 34 (3):370–374.

Akazawa, K., R. Okuno, *and* H. Kusumoto. 1999. Relation between intrinsic viscoelasticity and activation level of the human finger muscle during voluntary isometric contraction. *Frontiers of Medical and Biological Engineering* 9 (2):123–35.

Alexander, F.M. 1932. *The Use of Self*. London: Metheun & Co. Ltd.

Alter, M.J. 1997. *Sport Stretch*. Champaign, IL: Human Kinetics.

Alway, S.E. 1994. Force and contractile characteristics after stretch overload in quail anterior latissimus dorsi muscle. *Journal of Applied Physiology*. 77 (1):135–141.

Amako, M., T. Oda, K. Masuoka, et al. 2003. Effect of static stretching on prevention of injuries for military recruits. *Military Medicine* 168 (6):442–446.

American College of Sports Medicine. 2004. Position stand: exercise & hypertension. *Medicine & Science in Sports and Exercise* 36:533–553.

American College of Sports Medicine. 1998. The recommended quantity and quality of exercise for developing and maintaining cardiorespiratory and muscular fitness and flexibility in healthy adults. *Medicine & Science in Sports & Exercise* 30 (6):975–991.

Anderson, B., *and* E.R. Burke. 1991. Scientific, medical, and practical aspects of stretching. *Clinics in Sports Medicine* 10 (1):63–86.

Anderson, B. 2000. *Stretching*. Bolinas, Ca: Shelter Publications

Askling, C., H. Lund, T. Saartok, *and* A. Thorstensson. 2002. Self-reported hamstring injuries in student dancers. *Scandinavian Journal of Medicine & Science in Sports* 12:230–235.

Askling, C., T. Saartok, *and* A. Thorstensson. 2006. Type of acute hamstring strain affects flexibility, strength, and time to return to pre-injury level. *British Journal of Sports Medicine* 40:40–44.

Askling, C., M. Tengvar, T. Saartok, *and* A. Thorstensson. 2000. Sports related hamstring strains: two cases with different etiologies and injury sites. *Scandinavian Journal of Medicine & Science in Sports* 10:304–307.

Askling, C.M., M. Tengvar, T. Saartok, and A. Thorstensson. 2007. Acute first-time hamstring strains during slow-speed stretching: clinical, magnetic resonance imaging, and recovery characteristics. *American Journal of Sports Medicine* 35:1716–1724.

Babault, N., M. Pousson, A. Michaut, and J. Van Hoecke. 2003. Effect of quadriceps femoris muscle length on neural activation during isometric and concentric contractions. *Journal of Applied Physiology*. 94 (3):983–990.

Bagni, M.A., G. Cecchi, B. Colombini, et al. 2002. A non-cross-bridge stiffness in activated frog muscle fibers. *Biophysical Journal* 82:3118–3127.

Bandy, W.D., *and* J.M. Irion. 1994. The effect of time on static stretch on the flexibility of the hamstring muscles. *Physical Therapy* 74 (9):845–852.

Behm, D.G., A. Bambury, F. Cahill, et al. 2004. Effect of acute static stretching on force, balance, reaction time, and movement time. *Medicine & Science in Sports & Exercise* 36 (8):1397–1402.

Bixler, B.A., *and* R.L. Jones. 1992. High-school football injuries: effects of a post-halftime warm-up and stretching routine. The Family Practice Research Journal 12:131–139.

Black, J.D.J., M. Freeman, *and* E.D. Stevens. 2002. A 2 week routine stretching programme did not prevent contraction-induced injury in mouse muscle. *Journal of Physiology* 544(1):137–147.

Blair, S.N., H.W. Kohl III, *and* N.N. Goodyear. 1987. Relative risks for running and exercise injuries: studies in three populations. *Research Quarterly for Exercise and Sport* 58:221–228.

Bojsen-Moller, J., S.P. Magnusson, L.R. Rasmussen, *and* M. Kjaer, P. Aagaard. 2005. Muscle performance during maximal isometric and dynamic contractions is influenced by the stiffness of the tendinous structures. *Journal of Applied Physiology* 99 (3):986–994.

Borms, J., P. van Roy, J.P. Santens, et al. 1987. Optimal duration of static stretching exercises for improvement of coxo-femoral flexibility. *Journal of Sports Sciences* 5 (1):39–47.

Bosco, C., I. Tarkka, *and* P.V. Komi. 1982. Effect of elastic energy and myoelectrical potentiation of triceps surae during stretch-shortening cycle exercise. *International Journal of Sports Medicine* 3:137–140.

Braith, R.W., J.E. Graves, M.L. Pollock, et al. 1989. Comparison of two versus three days per week of variable resistance training during 10 and 18 week programs. *International Journal of Sports Medicine* 10:450–454.

Brockett, C.L., D.L. Morgan, *and* U. Proske. 2004. Predicting hamstring strain injury in elite athletes. *Medicine & Science in Sports & Exercise* 36:379–387.

Brooks, S.V., E. Zerba, *and* J.A. Faulkner. 1995. Injury to muscle fibers after single stretches of passive and maximally stimulated muscles in mice. *Journal of Physiology* 488:459–469.

Brunet, M.E., S.D. Cook, M.R. Brinker, et al. 1990. A survey of running injuries in 1505 competitive and recreational runners. *Journal of Sports Medicine and Physical Fitness* 30:307–315.

Buroker, K.C., *and* J.A. Schwane. 1989. Does postexercise static stretching alleviate delayed muscle soreness? *Physician Sportsmed* 17:65–83.

Butler, R.J., H.P. Crowell III, *and* I.M. Davis. 2003. Lower extremity stiffness: implications for performance and injury. *Clinical Biomechanics* 18:511–517.

Butterfield, T.A., *and* W. Herzog. 2006. Effect of altering starting length and activation timing of muscle on fiber strain and muscle damage. *Journal of Applied Physiology* 100 (5):1489–1498.

Chan, S.P., Y. Hong, *and* P.D. Robinson. 2001. Flexibility and passive resistance of the hamstrings of young adults using two different static protocols. *Scandinavian Journal of Medicine & Science in Sports* 11 (2):81–86.

Church, J.B., M.S. Wiggins, F.M. Moode, et al. 2001. Effect of warm-up and flexibility treatments on vertical jump performance. *Journal of Strength & Conditioning Research* 15 (3):332–336.

Coburn, J. W., et al. November 2004. Mechanomyographic responses of the vastus medialis to isometric and eccentric muscle actions. *Medicine & Science in Sports & Exercise* 36 (11):1916–1922.

Cocchiarella, L., and G.B.J. Andersson, eds. 2005. *Guides To The Evaluation Of Permanent Impairment.* Chicago: American Medical Association.

Condon, S.M., and R.S. Hutton. 1987. Soleus muscle electromyographic activity and ankle dorsiflexion range of motion during four stretching procedures. *Physical Therapy* 67 (1):24–40.

Conley, D.S., J.L. Belt, N.L. Hochstein, et al. Supp. May 2006. Proprioceptive neuromuscular facilitation but not static or ballistic stretching increases one repetition maximum bench press. *Medicine & Science in Sports & Exercise* 38:S295.

Corbin, C.B. 1984. Flexibility. *Clinics in Sports Medicine* 3:101–117.

Cornelius, W.L., K, Ebrahim, J, Watson, et al. 1992. The effects of cold application and modified PNF stretching techniques on hip joint flexibility in college males. *Research Quarterly for Exercise and Sport* 63:311–314.

Cornwell, A., A.G. Nelson, G.D. Heise, et al. 2001. Acute effects of passive muscle stretching on vertical jump performance. *Journal of Human Movement Studies* 40:307–324.

Craib, M.W., V.A. Mitchell, *and* K.B. Fields. 1996. The association between flexibility and running economy in sub-elite male runners. *Medicine & Science in Sports & Exercise* 28:737–743.

Cramer, J.T., T.J. Housh, G.O. Johnson, et al. 2004. Acute effects of static stretching on peak torque in women. *Journal of Strength & Conditioning Research* 18:236–241.

Cross K.M., and T.W. Worrell. 1999. Effects of a static stretching program on the incidence of lower extremity musculotendinous strains. *Journal of Athletic Training* 34:11–14.

Dadebo, B., J. White, *and* K.P. George. 2004. A survey of flexibility training protocols and hamstring strains in professional football clubs in England. *British Journal of Sports Medicine* 38:388–394.

Decoster, L.C., R.L. Scanlon, K.D. Horn, et al. 2004. Standing and supine hamstring stretching are equally effective. *Journal of Athletic Training* 39:330–334.

Doud, J.R., and J.M. Walsh. 1995. Muscle fatigue and muscle length interaction: effect on the EMG frequency components. *Electromyography and Clinical Neurophysiology* 35:331–339.

Edman, K.A.P., and C. Reggiani. 1984. Redistribution of sarcomere length during isometric contraction of frog muscle fibres and its relation to tension creep. *Journal of Physiology* 351:169–198.

Ekstrand, J., and J. Gillquist. 1982. The frequency of muscle tightness and injuries in soccer players. *American Journal of Sports Medicine* 10:75–78.

Ekstrand, J., J. Gillquist, and S. Liljedahl. 1983. Prevention of soccer injuries: supervision by doctor and physiotherapist. *American Journal of Sports Medicine* 11:116–120.

Ekstrand, J., J. Gillquist, M. Moller, et al. 1983. Incidence of soccer injuries and their relation to training and team success. *American Journal of Sports Medicine* 11:63–67.

Entyre B.R., and L.D. Abraham. 1986. Gains in range of ankle dorsiflexion using three popular stretching techniques. *American Journal of Sports Medicine* 65:189–196.

Entyre, B.R., and E.J. Lee. 1987. Comments on proprioceptive neuromuscular facilitation stretching techniques. *Research Quarterly for Exercise and Sport* 58:184–188.

Evetovich, T.K., N.J. Nauman, D.S. Conley , et al. Supp. May 2004. Effect of static stretching on torque, electro-mechanical delay, electro-torque delay, and electromechanical efficiency. *Medicine & Science in Sports & Exercise* 36:S343

Faigenbaum, A.D., M. Bellucci, A. Bernieri, et al. 2005. Acute effects of different warm-up protocols on fitness performance in children. *Journal of Strength & Conditioning Research* 19:376–381.

Fawcett, D.W. *Bloom and Fawcett: A textbook of histology*. 11th ed. 1986. Philadelphia: WB Saunders Co.

Fowles, J.R., D.G. Sale, *and* J.D. MacDougall. 2000. Reduced strength after passive stretch of the human plantar flexors. *Journal of Applied Physiology* 89:1179–1188.

Fukunaga, T., Y. Kawakami, K. Kubo, et al. 2002. Muscle and tendon interactions during human movements. *Exercise and Sport Sciences Review* 30:106–110.

Fürst, D.O., M. Osborn, R. Nave, et al. 1988. The organization of titin filaments in the half-sarcomere revealed by monoclonal antibodies in immunoelectron microscopy: a map of ten nonrepetitive epitopes starting at the Z line extends close to the M line. *Journal of Cell Biology* 106:1563–1572.

Gajdosik, R.L., M.A. Rieck, D.K. Sullivan, et al. 1993. Comparison of four clinical tests for assessing hamstring muscle length. *Journal of Orthopaedic and Sports Physical Therapy*:614–618.

Garrett, W.E., Jr. 1990. Muscle strain injuries: clinical and basic aspects. *Medicine & Science in Sports & Exercise* 22:436–443.

Garrett, W.E., Jr. 1996. Muscle strain injuries. *American Journal of Sports Medicine* 24:S2–8.

Garrett, W.E., M.R. Safran, A.V. Seaber, et al. 1987. Biomechanial comparison of stimulated and non-stimulated skeletal muscle pulled to failure. *American Journal of Sports Medicine* 15:448–454.

Girouard, C.K., and B.F. Hurley. 1995. Does strength training inhibit gains in range of motion from flexibility training in older adults? *Medicine & Science in Sports & Exercise* 27:1444–1449.

Gleim, G.W., *and* M.P. McHugh. 1997. Flexibility and its effects on sports injury and performance. *Sports Medicine* 24:289–299.

Gleim, G.W., N.S. Stachenfeld, *and* J.A. Nicholas. 1990. The influence of flexibility on the economy of walking and jogging. *Journal of Orthopaedic and Sports Physical Therapy* 8:814–823.

Godges, J.J., P.G. MacRae, *and* K. A. Engelke. 1993. Effects of exercise on hip range of motion, trunk muscle performance, and gait economy. *Physical Therapy* 73:468–477.

61. Godges, J.J., H. MacRae, C. Longdon, et al. 1989. The effects of two stretching procedures on hip range of motion and gait economy. *J. Orthop. Phys. Med.* 10:350–357.

Goldspink, D.F., V.M. Cox, S.K. Smith, et al. 1995. Muscle growth in response to mechanical stimuli. *American Journal of Physiology* 268: E288–297.

Granzier, H., and S. Labeit. 2002. Cardiac titin: an adjustable multi-functional spring. *Journal of Physiology* 541:335–342.

Graves, J.E., M.L. Pollock, A.E. Jones, et al. 1989. Specificity of limited range of motion variable resistance training. *Medicine & Science in Sports & Exercise* 21:84–89.

Halbertsma, J.P.K., and L.N.H. Goeken. 1994. Stretching exercises: effect on passive extensibility and stiffness in short hamstrings of healthy subjects. *Archives of Physical Medicine and Rehabilitation* 75:976–981.

Halbertsma, J.P., I. Mulder, L.N.H. Goeken, et al. 1999. Repeated passive stretching: acute effect on the passive muscle moment and extensibility of short hamstrings. *Archives of Physical Medicine and Rehabilitation* 80:407–414.

Halbertsma, J.P.K., A.I. van Bolhuis, *and* L.N.H. Goeken. 1996. Sport stretching: effect on passive muscle stiffness of short hamstrings. *Archives of Physical Medicine and Rehabilitation* 77:688–692.

Handel, M., T. Horstmann, H.H. Dickhuth, et al. 1997. Effects of contract-relax stretching training on muscle performance in athletes. *European Journal of Applied Physiology and Occupational Physioliology* 76:400–408.

Hartig, D.E., and J.M. Henderson. 1999. Increasing hamstring flexibility decreases lower extremity overuse injuries in military basic trainees. *American Journal of Sports Medicine* 27:173–176.

Hartley-O'Brien, S.J. 1990. Six mobilization exercises for active range of hip flexion. *Research Quarterly for Exercise and Sport* 51:625–635.

Helmer, K.G., J. Wellen, P. Grigg, et al. 2004. Measurement of the spatial redistribution of water in rabbit achilles tendon in response to static tensile loading. *Journal of Biomechanical Engineering* 126:651–656.

Helmes, M., K. Trombitas, *and* H. Granzier. 1996. Titin develops restoring force in rat cardiac myocytes. *Circulation Research* 79:619–626.

Henricson, A.S., K. Fredriksson, I. Persson, et al. 1984. The effect of heat and stretching on the range of hip motion. *Journal of Orthopaedic and Sports Physical Therapy* 6:110–115.

Herbert, R.D., and M. Gabriel. 2002. Effects of stretching before and after exercising on muscle soreness and risk of injury: a systematic review. *British Medical Journal* 325:468–470.

Herzog, W., R. Schachar, *and* T.R. Leonard. 2003. Characterization of the passive component of force enhancement following active stretching of skeletal muscle. *The Journal of Experimental Biology* 206:3635–3643.

Hewett, T.E., K.R. Ford, *and* G.D. Myer. 2006. Anterior cruciate ligament injuries in female athletes, part 2, a meta-analysis of neuromuscular interventions aimed at injury prevention. *American Journal of Sports Medicine* 34:490–498.

High, D.M., E.T. Howley, *and* B.D. Franks. 1989. The effects of static stretching and warm-up on prevention of delayed onset muscle soreness. *Research Quarterly for Exercise and Sport* 60:357–361.

Higuchi, H., T. Yoshioka, *and* K. Maruyama. 1988. Positioning of actin filaments and tension generation in skinned muscle fibres released after stretch beyond overlap of the actin and myosin filaments. *Journal of Muscle Research and Cell Motility* 9:491–498.

Hill, A.V. 1938. The heat of shortening and the dynamic constants of muscle. *Proceedings of the Royal Society of London.* 126:136–195.

Hilyer, J.C., K.C. Brown, A.T. Sirles, *and* L. Peoples. 1990. A flexibility intervention to reduce the incidence severity of joint injuries among municipal firefighters. *Journal of Occupational Medicine* 32:631–637.

Holmich, P., P. Uhrskou, L. Ulnits, et al. 1999. Active physical training for long-standing adductor-related groin pain. *Lancet* 353:439–443.

Holt, J., L.E. Holt, *and* T.W. Pelhan. 1996. Flexibility redefined. In *XIIIth International Symposium for Biomechanics in Sport*, ed. T. Bauer, 170–174. Ontario: Lakehead University.

Horowits, R., *and* R.J. Podolsky. 1987. The positional stability of thick filaments in activated skeletal muscle depends on sarcomere length: evidence for the role of titin filaments. *Journal of Cell Biology* 105:2217–2223.

Horowits, R., E.S. Kempner, M.E. Hisher, et al. 1986. A physiological role for titin and nebulin in skeletal muscle. *Nature* 323:160–164.

Hortobagyi, T., J. Faludi, J. Tihanyi, et al. 1985. Effects of intense stretching-flexibility training on the mechanical profile of the knee extensors and on the range of motion of the hip joint. *International Journal of Sports Medicine* 6:317–321.

Howell, D.W. 1984. Musculoskeletal profile and incidence of musculoskeletal injuries in lightweight, women rowers. *American Journal of Sports Medicine* 12:278–282.

Hunter, J.P., and R.N. Marshall. 2002. Effects of power and flexibility training on vertical jump technique. *Medicine & Science in Sports & Exercise* 34:478–486.

Hutton, R.S., and S.W. Atwater. 1992. Acute and chronic adaptations of muscle proprioceptors in response to increased use. *Sports Medicine* 14:406–412.

Huxley, A.F. 1957. Muscle structure and theories of contraction. *Progress in Biophysics and Biophysical Chemistry* 7:255–318.

Huxley, A.F., and R.M. Simmons. 1971. Mechanical properties of the cross-bridges of frog striated muscle. *Journal of Physiology* 218:59–60.

Ingraham, S.J. 2003. The role of flexibility in injury prevention and athletic performance: Have we stretched the truth? *Minnesota Medicine* 86:58–61.

Ito, M., Y. Kawakami, Y. Ichinose, et al. 1998. Nonisometric behavior of fascicles during isometric contractions of a human muscle. *Journal of Applied Physiology* 85:1230–1235.

Jacobs, J.V., F.B. Horak, V.K. Tran, et al. 2006. Multiple balance tests improve the assessment of postural stability in subjects with Parkinson's disease. *Journal of Neurology, Neurosurgery & Psychiatry* 77:322–326.

Jacobs, S.J., *and* B.L. Berson. 1986. Injuries to runners: a study of entrants to a 10,000 meter race. *American Journal of Sports Medicine* 14:151–155.

Jobe, F.W., D.R. Moynes, J.E. Tibone, et al. 1984. An EMG analysis of the shoulder in pitching. A second report. *American Journal of Sports Medicine* 12:218–220.

Johansson, P.H., L. Lindstrom, G. Sundelin, et al. 1999. The effects of pre-exercise stretching on muscle soreness, tenderness and force loss following heavy eccentric exercise. *Scandinavian Journal of Medicine & Science in Sports* 9:219–225.

Jones, B.H., D.N. Cowan, J.P. Tomlinson, et al. 1993. Epidemiology of injuries associated with physical training among young men in the army. *Medicine & Science in Sports & Exercise* 25:197–203.

Jones, B.H., and J.J. Knapik. 1999. Physical training and exercise-related injuries. Surveillance, research and injury prevention in military populations. *Sports Medicine* 27:111–125.

Jonhagen, S., G. Nemeth, *and* E. Eriksson. 1994. Hamstring injuries in sprinters. The role of concentric and eccentric hamstring muscle strength and flexibility. *American Journal of Sports Medicine* 22:262–266.

Jonsson, E., A. Seiger, *and* H. Hirschfeld. 2004. One-leg stance in healthy young and elderly adults: a measure of postural steadiness? *Clinical Biomechanics* 19:688–694.

Julian, F.J., *and* D.L. Morgan. 1979. Intersarcomere dynamics during fixed-end tetanic contractions of frog muscle fibers. *Journal of Physiology* 293:365–378.

Julian, F.J., and D.L. Morgan. 1979. The effect of tension of non-uniform distribution of length changes applied to frog muscle fibres. *Journal of Physiology* 293:379–393.

Kerrigan, D.C., A. Xenopoulos-Oddsson, M.J. Sullivan, et al. 2003. Effect of a hip flexor-stretching program on gait in the elderly. *Archives of Physical Medicine and Rehabilitation* 84:1–6.

Kibler, W.B., C. Goldberg, *and* T.J. Chandler. 1991. Functional biomechanical deficits in running athletes with plantar fasciitis. *American Journal of Sports Medicine* 266:185–196.

Kirby, R. L., F.C. Simms, V.J. Symington, et al. 1981. Flexibility and musculoskeletal symptomatology in female gymnasts and age-matched controls. *American Journal of Sports Medicine* 9:160–164.

Klinge, K., S.P. Magnusson, E.B. Simonsen, et al. 1997. The effect of strength and flexibility training on skeletal muscle electromyographic activity, stiffness, and viscoelastic stress relaxation response. *American Journal of Sports Medicine* 25:710–716.

Knudson, D., K. Bennett, R. Corn, et al. 2001. Acute effects of stretching are not evident in the kinematics of the vertical jump. *Journal of Strength & Conditioning Research* 15:98–101.

Knudson, D.V., P. Magnusson, *and* M. McHugh. 2000. Current issues in flexibility fitness. *President's Council on Physical Fitness and Sports* 3:1–6.

Knudson, D.V., G.J. Noffal, R.E. Bahamonde, et al. 2004. Stretching has no effect on tennis serve performance. *Journal of Strength & Conditioning Research* 18:654–656.

Kokkonen, J., A.G. Nelson, *and* A. Cornwell. 1998. Acute muscle stretching inhibits maximal strength performance. *Research Quarterly for Exercise and Sport* 69:411–415.

Kokkonen, J., A.G. Nelson, C. Eldredge, J.B. Winchester. 2007. Chronic Static Stretching Improves Exercise Performance. *Medicine & Science in Sports & Exercise* 39(10):1825–1831.

Krabak, B.J., E.R. Laskowski, M.J. Stuart, et al. 2001. Neurophysiological influences on hamstring flexibility: a pilot study. *Clinical Journal of Sport Medicine* 11:241–246.

Kubo, K., H. Kanehisa, *and* T. Fukunaga. 2002. Effect of stretching training on the viscoelastic properties of human tendon structures in vivo. *Journal of Applied Physiology* 92:595–601.

Kurokawa, S., T. Fukunaga, *and* S. Fukashiro. 2001. Behavior of fascicles and tendinous structures of human gastrocnemius during vertical jumping. *Journal of Applied Physiology* 90:1349–1358.

Lally, D.A. Stretching and injury in distance runners. Supp. 1994. *Medicine & Science in Sports & Exercise* 26 473.

Lange, S., F.Q. Xiang, A. Yakovenko, et al. 2005. The kinase domain of titin controls muscle gene expression and protein turnover. *Science* 308:1599–1603.

LaRoche, D.P., *and* D.A.J. Connolly. 2006. Effects of stretching on passive muscle tension and response to eccentric exercise. *American Journal of Sports Medicine* 34:1000–1007.

Leach, R.E., S. James, *and* S. Wasilewski. 1981. Achilles tendinitis. *American Journal of Sports Medicine* 9:93–98.

Lee, E.J., B.R. Etnyre, H.B.W. Poindexter, et al. 1989. Flexibility characteristics of elite female and male volleyball players. *Journal of Sports Medicine and Physical Fitness* 29:49–51.

Linke, W.A. 2000. Stretching molecular springs: elasticity of titin filaments in vertebrate striated muscle. *Histology and Histopathology* 15:799–811.

Linke, W.A. 2004. Multiple sources of passive stress relaxation in muscle fibres. *Physics in Medicine and Biology.* 49:3613–3627.

Lucas, R.C., and R. Koslow. 1984. Comparative study of static, dynamic, and proprioceptive neuromuscular facilitation stretching techniques on flexibility. *Perceptual and Motor Skills* 58:615–618.

Macera, C.A., R.R. Pate, K.E. Powell, et al. 1989. Predicting lower-extremity injuries among habitual runners. *Archives of Internal Medicine* 149:2565–2568.

Macpherson, P.C.D., M.A. Schork, *and* J.A. Faulkner. 1996. Contraction-induced injury to single fiber segments from fast and slow muscles of rats by single stretches. *American Journal of Physiology* 271:1438–1446.

Maffiuletti, N.A., and A. Martin. 2001. Progressive versus rapid rate of contraction during 7 wk of isometric resistance training. *Medicine & Science in Sports & Exercise* 33:1220–1227.

Magid, A., and D.J. Law. 1985. Myofibrils bear most of the resting tension in frog skeletal muscle. *Science* 230:1280–1282.

Magnusson, S.P. 1998. Passive properties of human skeletal muscle during stretch maneuvers. A review. *Scandinavian Journal of Medicine & Science in Sports* 8:65–77.

Magnusson, S.P., P. Aagaard, B. Larsson, et al. 1996. Passive energy absorption by human muscle-tendon unit is unaffected by increase in intramuscular temperature. *Journal of Applied Physiology* 88:1215–1220.

Magnusson, S.P., P. Aagaard, *and* J.J. Nielson. 2000. Passive energy return after repeated stretches of the hamstring muscle-tendon unit. *Medicine & Science in Sports & Exercise* 32:1160–1164.

Magnusson, S.P., E.B. Simonsen, P. Aagaard, et al. 1996. Mechanical and physical responses to stretching with and without preisometric contraction in human skeletal muscle. *Archives of Physical Medicine and Rehabilitation* 77:373–378.

Magnusson, S.P., E.B. Simonsen, P. Aagaard, et al. 1996. A mechanism for altered flexibility in human skeletal muscle. *Journal of Physiology* 497:291–298.

Mahieu, N.N., E. Witvrouw, V. Stevens, et al. 2006. Intrinsic risk factors for the development of achilles tendon overuse injury. *American Journal of Sports Medicine* 34:226–235.

Mair, S.D., A.V. Seaber, R.R. Glisson, et al. 1996. The role of fatigue in susceptibility to acute muscle strain injury. *American Journal of Sports Medicine* 24:137–143.

Malliaropoulos, N., S. Papalexandris, A. Papalada, et al. 2004. The role of stretching in rehabilitation of hamstring injuries: 80 athletes follow-up. *Medicine & Science in Sports & Exercise* 36:756–759.

Markos, P.D. 1979. Ipsilateral and contralateral effects of proprioceptive neuromuscular facilitation techniques on hip motion and electromyographic activity. *Physical Therapy* 59:1366–1373.

McGuine, T.A., and J.S. Keene. 2006. The effect of a balance training program on the risk of ankle sprains in high school athletes. *American Journal of Sports Medicine* 34:1103–1111.

McKay, G.D., P.A. Goldie, W.R. Payne, et al. 2001. Ankle injuries in basketball: injury rate and risk factors. *British Journal of Sports Medicine* 35:103–108.

McHugh, M.P., D.A.J. Connolly, R.G. Eston, et al. 1999. The role of passive stiffness in symptoms of exercise-induced muscle damage. *American Journal of Sports Medicine* 27:594–599.

McHugh, M.P., I.J. Kremenic, M.B. Fox, et al. Supp. May 1996. The relationship of linear stiffness of human muscle to maximum joint range of motion. *Medicine & Science in Sports & Exercise* 28:77

McHugh, M.P., I.J. Kremenic, M.B. Fox, et al. 1998. The role of mechanical and neural restraints to joint range of motion during passive stretch. *Medicine & Science in Sports & Exercise* 30:928–932.

McHugh, M.P., R. Roy, and D.T. Tetro. Supp. May 2001. Does stretch-induced torque augmentation reflect crossbridge stiffness? *Medicine & Science in Sports & Exercise* 33:186

McHugh, M.P., and D.T. Tetro. Supp. May 2002. A mechanism for the repeated bout effect? *Medicine & Science in Sports & Exercise* 34:184

McMillian, D.J., J.H. Moore, B.S. Hatler, et al. 2006. Dynamic vs. static-stretching warm up: The effect on power and agility performance. *Journal of Strength & Conditioning Research* 20:492–499.

McNeal, J.R., and W.A. Sands. 2006. Stretching for performance enhancement. *Current Sports Medicine Reports* 5:141–146.

Millar, P.J., S.R Bray, M.J. MacDonald, and N. McCartney. 2008. The hypotensive effects of isometric handgrip training using an inexpensive spring handgrip training device. *Journal of Cardiopulmonary Rehabilitation and Prevention* 28(3):203–7.

Mitchell, U.H., J.W. Myrer, J.T. Hopkins, et al. Supp. May 2006. Reciprocal inhibition, successive inhibition, autogenic inhibition, or stretch perception alteration: Why do PNF stretches work? *Medicine & Science in Sports & Exercise* 38:66

Miyahara, Y., Y. Ogura, H. Naito, et al. Supp. May 2005. Effect of proprioceptive neuromuscular facilitation stretching and static stretching on maximal voluntary contraction. *Medicine & Science in Sports & Exercise* 37:441

Moller, M., J. Ekstrand, B. Oberg, et al. 1985. Duration of stretching effect on range of motion in lower extremities. *Archives of Physical Medicine and Rehabilitation* 66:171–173.

Morgan, D.L., and U. Proske. 2004. Popping sarcomere hypothesis explains stretch-induced muscle damage. *Clinical and Experimental Pharmacology & Physiology* 31:541–545.

Moore, M.A., and R.S. Hutton. 1980. Electromyographic investigation of muscle stretching techniques. *Medicine & Science in Sports & Exercise* 12:322–329.

Myers, J.B., K.G. Laudner, M.R. Pasquale, et al. 2006. Glenohumeral range of motion deficits and posterior shoulder tightness in throwers with pathologic internal impingement. *American Journal of Sports Medicine* 34:385–391.

Nelson, A.G., J. Kokkonen, and D.A. Arnall. 2005. Acute muscle stretching inhibits muscle strength endurance performance. *Journal of Strength & Conditioning Research* 19:338–343.

Nelson, A.G., J. Kokkonen, C. Eldredge, et al. 2001. Chronic stretching and running economy. *Scandinavian Journal of Medicine & Science in Sports* 11:260–265.

Nesse, M., and M.P. McHugh. Supp. May 2006. The effect of static stretching on strength loss and pain following eccentric exercise. *Medicine & Science in Sports & Exercise* 38:387

Noback, C.R., N.L. Strominger, and R.J. Demarest, eds. 1996. *The Human Nervous System: Structure and Function.* 5th ed. Baltimore: Williams & Wilkins.

Noffal, G., D. Knudson, and L. Brown. Supp. May 2004. Effects of stretching the upper limb on throwing speed and isokinetic shoulder torques. *Medicine & Science in Sports & Exercise* 36:136–137

Noonan, T.J., T.M. Best, A.V. Seaber, et al. 1993. Thermal effects on skeletal muscle tensile behavior. *American Journal of Sports Medicine* 21:517–522.

Nosaka, K., and P.M. Clarkson. 1997. Influence of previous concentric exercise on eccentric exercise-induced muscle damage. *Journal of Sports Sciences* 15:477–483.

O'Loughllin, J. 1993. Incidence of and risk factors for falls and injurious falls among the community-dwelling elderly. *American Journal of Epidemiology* 137:342–354.

Olsen, O.E., G. Myklebust, L. Engebretsen, et al. 2004. Injury mechanisms for anterior cruciate ligament injuries in team handball. *American Journal of Sports Medicine* 32:1002–1005.

Olsen, O.E., G. Myklebust, L. Engebretsen, et al. 2005. Exercises to prevent lower limb injuries in youth sports: cluster randomised controlled trial. *British Medical Journal* 26; 330:449.

Orchard, J. 2002. Biomechanics of muscle strain injury. *New Zealand Journal of Medicine* 30:92–98.

Osternig, L.R., R. Robertson, R. Troxel, et al. 1987. Muscle activation during proprioceptive neuromuscular facilitation (PNF) stretching techniques. *American Journal of Physical Medicine* 66:298–307.

Pastanga, N., D. Field, and R. Soames. 994. *Anatomy and Human Movement.* Oxford: Butterworth-Heinemann.

Pilates, J.H. 1945. *Return to Life through Contrology.* Incline Village, Ne: J.J. Augustin.

Pinnington, H.C., D.G. Lloyd, T.F. Besier, et al. 2005. Kinematic and electromyography analysis of submaximal differences running on a firm surface compared with soft, dry sand. *European Journal of Applied Physiology* 94:242–253.

Pope, R.P., R. Herbert, and J. Kirwan. 1998. Effects of ankle dorsiflexion range and pre-exercise calf muscle stretching on injury risk in Army recruits. *Australian Journal of Physiotherapy* 44:165–172,

Pope, R.P., R.D. Herbert, J.D. Kirwan, et al. 2000. A randomized trial of pre-exercise stretching for prevention of lower-limb injury. *Medicine & Science in Sports & Exercise* 32:271–277.

Power, K., D. Behm, F. Cahill, et al. 2004. An acute bout of static stretching: effects on force and jumping performance. *Medicine & Science in Sports & Exercise* 36:1389–1396.

Prentice, W.E. 1983. A comparison of static stretching and PNF stretching for improving hip joint flexibility. *Athletic Training* 18:56–59.

Preetha, N., G.W. Yimin, M. Helmes, et al. 2005. Restoring force development by titin/connectin and assessment of Ig domain unfolding. *Journal of Muscle Research and Cell Motility* 26:307–317.

Raab D.M., J.C. Agre, M. McAdam, et al. 1988. Light resistance and stretching exercise in elderly women: effect upon flexibility. *Archives of Physical Medicine and Rehabilitation* 69:268–272.

Ray, C.A., and D.I. Carrasco. 2000. Isometric handgrip training reduces arterial pressure at rest without changes in sympathetic nerve activity. *American Journal of Physiology. Heart and Circulatory Physiology* 279:H245–H249.

Reid, D.C., R.S. Burnham, L.A. Saboe, et al. 1987. Lower extremity flexibility patterns in classical ballet dancers and their correlation to lateral hip and knee injuries. *American Journal of Sports Medicine* 15:347–352.

Reid, D.A., and P.J. McNair. 2004. Passive force, angle, and stiffness changes after stretching of hamstring muscles. *Medicine & Science in Sports & Exercise* 36:1944–1948.

Roberts, J.M., and K. Wilson. 1999. Effect of stretching duration on the active and passive range of motion in the lower extremity. *British Journal of Sports Medicine* 33:259–263.

Rodenburg, J., D. Steenbeek, P. Schiereck, et al. 1994. Warm-up stretching and massage diminish harmful effects of eccentric exercise. *International Journal of Sports Medicine* 15:414–419.

Ross, J. 1999. Effect of lower-extremity position at stretching on hamstring muscle flexibility. *Journal of Strength & Conditioning Research* 13:124–129.

Rowlands, A.V., V.F. Marginson, J. Lee. 2003. Chronic flexibility gains: effect of isometric contraction duration during proprioceptive neuromuscular facilitation stretching techniques. *Research Quarterly for Exercise and Sport* 74:47–51.

Ryan, E.E., R. Lopez, R.M. Rossi, et al. Supp. May 2006. The effects of contract-relax-antagonist-contract form of PNF stretching on postural stability. *Medicine & Science in Sports & Exercise* 38:448

Sady, S.P., M. Wortman, and D. Blanke. 1982. Flexibility training: ballistic, static or proprioceptive neuromuscular facilitation? *Archives of Physical Medicine and Rehabilitation* 63:261–263

Safran, M.R., A.V. Seaber, and W.E. Garret, Jr. 1989. Warm-up and muscular injury prevention: an update. *Sports Medicine* 8:239–249.

Safran, M.R., W.E. Garrett, A.V. Seaber, et al. 1988. The role of warmup in muscular injury prevention. *American Journal of Sports Medicine* 16:123–129.

Schenck, R.C. Jr., ed. 1999. *Athletic Training and Sports Medicine.* 3rd ed. Rosemont, IL: American Academy of Orthopaedic Surgeons.

Schenkman, M.K., M. Shipp, J. Chandler, et al. 1996. Relationships between mobility of axial structures and physical performance. *Physical Therapy* 76:276–285.

Sherry, M.A., and T.M. Best. 2004. A comparison of 2 rehabilitation programs in the treatment of acute hamstring strains. *Journal of Orthopaedic and Sports Physical Therapy* 34:116–125.

Shellock, F.G., and W.E. Prentice. Warming-up and stretching for improved physical performance and prevention of sports-related injuries. *Sports Medicine* 2:267–278, 1985.

Shrier, I. 1999. Stretching before exercise does not reduce the risk of local muscle injury: a critical review of the clinical and basic science literature. *Clinical Journal of Sports Medicine* 9:221–227.

Shrier, I. 2004. Does stretching improve performance: a systematic and critical review of the literature. *Clinical Journal of Sport Medicine* 14:267–273.

Shrier, I, and K. Gossal. 2000. Myths and truths of stretching: individualized recommendations for healthy muscles. *The Physician and Sportsmedicine* 28:57–63.

Sinkjar, T., E. Toft, S. Andreassen, et al. 1988. Muscle stiffness in human ankle dorsiflexors: intrinsic and reflex components. *Journal of Neuroscience* 60:1110–1121.

Soderberg, G.L. 1997. *Kinesiology: Application to Pathological Motion.* Baltimore: Williams & Wilkins.

Song, H., K. Nakazato, and H. Nakajima. 2004. Effect of increased excursion of the ankle on the severity of acute eccentric contraction-induced strain injury of the gastrocnemius. *American Journal of Sports Medicine* 32:1263–1269.

Spencer, S.J., W.L. Cornelius, and D.W. Hill. Supp. May 1998. Concentric and isometric actions in proprioceptive neuromuscular facilitation stretching techniques. *Medicine & Science in Sports & Exercise* 30:164

Stephens, J., J. Davidson, J. DeRosa, et al. 2006. Lengthening the hamstring muscles without stretching using "awareness through movement". *Physical Therapy* 86:1641–1650.

Tanigawa, M.C. 1972. Comparison of the hold-relax procedure and passive mobilization on increasing muscle length. *Physical Therapy* 52:725–735.

Taylor, A.C., N. McCartney, M.V. Kamath, et al. 2003. Isometric training lowers resting blood pressure and modulates autonomic control. *Medicine & Science in Sports & Exercise* 35:251–256.

Taylor, D.C., D.E. Brooks, and J.B. Ryan. 1997. Viscoelastic characteristics of muscle: passive stretching versus muscular contractions. *Medicine & Science in Sports & Exercise* 29:1619–1624.

Taylor, D.C., J.D. Dalton, Jr., A.V. Seaber, et al. 1990. Viscoelastic properties of muscle-tendon units. The biomechanical effects of stretching. *American Journal of Sports Medicine* 18:300–309.

Thacker, S.B., D.F. Stroup, C.M. Branche, et al. 2003. Prevention of knee injuries in sports. A systematic review of the literature. *Journal of Sports Medicine and Physical Fitness.* 43:165–179.

Thacker, S.B., J. Gilchrist, D.F. Stroup, et al. 2004. The impact of stretching on sports injury risk: A systematic review of the literature. *Medicine & Science in Sports & Exercise* 36:371–378.

Toft, E., G.T. Espersen, S. Kalund, et al. 1989. Passive tension of the ankle before and after stretching. *American Journal of Sports Medicine* 17:489–494.

Tsuda, E., Y. Okamura, H. Otsuka, et al. 2001. Direct evidence of anterior cruciate ligament-hamstring reflex arc in humans. *American Journal of Sports Medicine* 29:83–87.

Tyler, T.F., S.J. Nicholas, R.J. Campbell, et al. 2001. The association of hip strength and flexibility with the incidence of adductor muscle strains in professional hockey players. *American Journal of Sports Medicine* 29:124–127.

Ussher M., R. West, R. Doshi, and A.K. Sampuran. 2006. Acute effect of isometric exercise on desire to smoke and tobacco withdrawal symptoms. Human Psychopharmacology 21 (1):39–46.

Van Mechelen, W., H. Hlobil, H.C.G. Kemper, et al. 1993. Prevention of running injuries by warm-up, cool-down, and stretching exercises. *American Journal of Sports Medicine* 21:711–719.

Wallmann, H.W., J.A. Mercer, and J.W. McWhorter. 2005. Surface electromyographic assessment of the effect of static stretching of the gastrocnemius on vertical jump performance. *Journal of Strength & Conditioning Research* 19:684–688.

Walter, S.D., L.E. Hart, J.M. McIntosh, et al. 1989. The Ontario cohort study of running-related injuries. *Archives of Internal Medicine* 149:2561–2564.

Wedderkopp, N., M. Kaltoft, B. Lundgaard, et al. 1999. Prevention of injuries in young female players in European team handball. A prospective intervention study. *Scandinavian Journal of Medicine & Science in Sports* 9:41–47.

Weerapong, P., P.A. Hume, and G.S. Kolt. Supp. May 2004. Warm-up, stretching, and massage before exercise: effects on passive stiffness and delayed-onset muscle soreness. *Medicine & Science in Sports & Exercise* 36:16

Weldon, S.M., and R.H. Hill. 2003. The efficacy of stretching for prevention of exercise-related injury: a systematic review of the literature. *Manual Therapy* 8:141–150.

Wessel, J., and A. Wan. 1994. Effect of stretching on the intensity of delayed-onset muscle soreness. *Clinical Journal of Sports Medicine* 4:83–87.

Whaley, W.H. et al., eds. *American College of Sports Medicine's Guidelines for Exercise Testing and Prescription.* 7th ed. 2006. Baltimore, Md: Lippincott Williams & Wilkins.

Wiktorsson-Moller, M., B. Oberg, J. Ekstrand, et al. 1983. Effects of warming up, massage, and stretching on range of motion and muscle strength in the lower extremity. *American Journal of Sports Medicine* 11:249–252.

Wilber, C.A., G.J. Holland, R.E. Madison, et al. 1995. An epidemiological analysis of overuse injuries among recreational cyclists. *International Journal of Sports Medicine* 16:201–206.

Wilmore, J.H., and D.L. Costill. *Physiology of Sport and Exercise.* Human Kinetics. Champaign, IL, 2005.

Wilson, G.J., B.C. Elliott, and G.A. Wood. 1992. Stretch shorten cycle performance enhancement through flexibility training. *Medicine & Science in Sports & Exercise* 24:116–123.

Winters, M.V., C.G. Blake, J.S. Trost, et al. 2004. Passive versus active stretching of hip flexor muscles in subjects with limited hip extension: a randomized clinical trial. *Physical Therapy* 84:800–807.

Witvrouw, E., J. Bellemans, R. Lysens, et al. 2001. Intrinsic risk factors for the development of patellar tendinitis in an athletic population. *American Journal of Sports Medicine* 29:190–195.

Witvrouw, E., L. Danneels, P. Asselman, et al. 2003. Muscle flexibility as a risk factor for developing muscle injuries in male professional soccer players. *American Journal of Sports Medicine* 31:41–46.

Woo, S.L.-Y., and J.A. Buckwalter, eds. *Injury and Repair of the Musculoskeletal Soft Tissues.* Symposium of the American Academy of Orthopaedic Surgeons, 1987.

Worrell, T.W. . 1994. Factors associated with hamstring injuries: an approach to treatment and preventative measures. *Sports Medicine* 17:335–345.

Worrell, T.W., T.L. Smith, and J. Winegardner. 1994. Effect of hamstring stretching on hamstring muscle performance. *Journal of Orthopaedic and Sports Physical Therapy Physical Therapy* 20:154–159.

Wright, R.W., K. Steger-May, B.L. Wasserlauf, et al. 2006. Elbow range of motion in professional baseball pitchers. *American Journal of Sports Medicine* 34:190–193.

Yang, S., M. Alnaqeeb, H. Simpson, et al. 1997. Changes in muscle fibre type, muscle mass and IGF-I gene expression in rabbit skeletal muscle subjected to stretch. *Journal of Anatomy* 190:613–22.

Yarrow, J.F., and T.W. Burns. May 2004. Supp. Static stretching inhibits maximal muscle endurance. *Medicine & Science in Sports & Exercise* 36:353

J. Ylinen, et al. 2003. Active neck muscle training in the treatment of chronic neck pain in women: a randomized controlled trial. *The Journal of the American Medical Association* 289 (19):2509–2516.

Young, W.B., and D.G. Behm. 2003. Effects of running, static stretching and practice jumps on explosive force production and jumping performance. *Journal of Sports Medicine and Physical Fitness* 43:21–27.

Zou, P., N. Pinotsis, S. Lange, Y.H. Song, et al. 2006. Anchoring of the giant muscle protein titin in muscle cells. *Nature* 439:229.